The
SECRET SOURCE
of Your Good Health

The
SECRET SOURCE
of Your Good Health

Chris Woollams
M.A. (Oxon)

And how it is linked to Allergies, Alzheimer's,
Asthma, Arthritis, Autism, Blood Pressure, Cancer,
Colitis, Constipation, Crohn's disease, Dementia,
Diabetes, Eczema, Hay fever, Heart Disease, IBS,
Multiple Sclerosis, Obesity, Parkinson's, Strokes,
Wheezing and, of course, Longevity.

First published in February 2014 by Health Issues Ltd

Cover design by Jeremy Baker.

ISBN 978-0-9565391-6-8

Second Edition: July 2014

Printed in England by CPI Group (UK) Ltd, Croydon CR04YY.
And printed in Australia by Griffin Press, Adelaide.

*For the American Professor of Rheumatism
and Arthritis who I met in the queue at
Dubai International airport.*

*For Larry and Jane, and Wendy and Jeremy.
Thanks for your help.*

Important Notice

This short info-book represents a review and an interpretation of a vast number of varied sources available to anyone on the subject of the microbiome.

Whilst the author has made every effort to ensure that the facts, information and conclusions are accurate and as up to date as possible at the time of publication, the author and publisher assume no responsibility.

The author is neither a fully qualified Health Practitioner nor a Doctor of Medicine and so is not qualified to give any advice on any medical matters. Many illnesses like cancer, Alzheimer's and diabetes are very serious and very individual diseases and readers must consult with experts and specialists in the appropriate medical field before taking, or refraining from taking, any action.

This book and the advice contained in it are not intended as an alternative to such specialist advice, which should be sought for accurate diagnosis and before any course of treatment.

The author and the publisher cannot be held responsible for any action, or lack of action, that is taken by any reader as a result of information contained in the text of this book. Such action is taken entirely at the reader's own risk.

*"I'll get by with
a little help from my friends"*

Richard Starkey (Ringo Starr) MBE

FOREWORD

Health is harmony of mind, body and spirit, according to the World Health Organisation (adapted). Every farmer, and every gardener knows that long term the health of crops, and the beauty in a garden come about from attention to the soil and the environment. We poison the soil of our fields and gardens at our peril.

Yet few of us in the 21st Century choose to be aware that every human body has its own inner garden of bacteria – the microbiome inside our intestines. Seven trillion cells of bacteria, the vast majority of them friendly and beneficial to our health, adapted and living with us to mutual benefit. They break down some foods so we can digest them, produce vitamins and other health giving substances, and help us remain healthy.

Louis Pasteur, the father of immunization, carries a heavy burden of guilt, despite all the benefits from his work – for colluding with us all in thinking "them and us" where "them" is the enemy. Antibiotics kill "them" (the bad guys) – but unfortunately also kill all the good guys (part of us that we need to thrive and survive). From this thinking, the whole of medicine uses 'antis' – anti-hypertensives, anti-inflammatories, anti-biotics, anti-cancer, anti-arthritic drugs. Against this, Claude Bernard, the other great 19th Century French medical giant, upheld the importance of the health of the soil.

On his death-bed Pasteur said *'Bernard avait raison; le microbe n'est rien, c'est le terrain qui est tout'*. ('Bernard was right; the microbe is nothing, it is the soil that's everything') – but contemporary medical practice has yet to catch up with Pasteur's new insight.

The beauty of Pasteur's approach is that we can blame 'them' rather than take responsibility for 'us'. In the 21st Century our biggest challenge is to take responsibility for ourselves (rather than seek a magic external bullet, or let other people control the food we eat), learn about the ways of health, and practice them wisely.

Chris Woollams does us a great service in clarifying this truth for our guts and for the food we eat. He points out the great volume of research that shows that 'loving our guts' and feeding the microbiome correctly is crucial in long term health and avoiding degenerative diseases. Never a word so true as "You are what you eat".

Dr Andrew Tresidder
MBBS MRCGP 1989 Cert Med Ed

CONTENTS

INTRODUCTION

So, there I was, standing at Immigration in Dubai International Airport. Unusually, there was a very, very long queue. Behind me was a shortish, elderly gentleman (by that I mean older than me), and we got chatting. He was a Professor of Rheumatism and Arthritis at his University Medical School in America. I told him that I was founder and editor of a holistic cancer charity that now had the biggest website in the UK. We compared notes; we had so much in common. We started to talk about bioactive compounds and drugs. *"We don't treat rheumatism with drugs anymore"*, he told me. *"They don't work and more often than not, make matters worse. We do it all with diet nowadays and the results are much better"*. Music to my ears.

We talked throughout the hour of waiting; four lines of people listened avidly as we swapped stories and facts. As we reached the moment to have our passports stamped, he said to me *"I bet you don't know about the Microbiome?"* I bet I do, and I told him!

His final words were simple but hugely important. And exactly as I have noted in articles I have previously written: *"The microbiome has a lot of top doctors and oncologists really worried in America. You cannot get better until it gets better, and they now know their treatments make matters worse"*.

I first wrote on this subject in 2006. The microbiome? Let me explain ...

CHAPTER 1

WHY YOU SHOULD BE HAPPY THAT YOUR TWO YEAR OLD CHILD HAS ANOTHER COLD

'She's got another cold. I don't understand it. I'd better take her to the doctor. She had one last week, and another only a couple of weeks ago. She's always getting colds. There must be something wrong with her'.

How many times have you heard this sort of commentary? The Doctor can't do much to help. Four colds in five weeks. He has cough mixture on hand; even antibiotics if the cold goes to her chest with an infection. Sadly, this 'solution' might only make matters worse.

You see, she hasn't got a cold. Sophie lives near a farm. This week, little 'Sophie' patted the dog and then, ten minutes later, she put her fingers in her mouth. Last week, the wind blew strongly from the cow sheds towards her open bedroom window. The week before? That time she held a new chick.

'Why do kids who live outdoors in the fresh air seem to get so many colds? You would have thought it would be the opposite'. We've heard this said too.

The crucial point is that the runny nose, the slight cough and the temperature are the best things that can happen to Sophie. She doesn't have a cold. Instead she is building an immune system fit to last a lifetime and protect her from all manner of diseases.

Exposure

In the *New England Journal of Medicine* (Feb 24th 2011) German researchers led by Markus J. Ege, MD, of the University Children's Hospital, Munich showed that school-aged children who lived on farms were between 30 and 50 per cent less likely to have asthma than non-farm children who lived in towns nearby.

The study was developed to test a theory that had been gathering momentum; namely, that exposure to a wide range of microbes is crucial to the development of a strong immune system.

There is little doubt that farm-dwelling children are exposed to more bacteria and fungi than other children and one possible 'cause' of asthma has been dubbed 'The hygiene hypothesis'. According to the hypothesis, exposure to bacteria and fungi from environmental sources early in life protects against asthma and other allergies by helping the immune system to develop fully. The corollary also seems to apply – that increasingly clean and sanitised urban environments may at least partially explain why asthma rates have doubled in developed nations in just the last three decades.

In the German study, the researchers conducted DNA analysis on dust samples taken from mattresses of two groups of children (farm dwellers and city dwellers). They also analysed settled dust samples taken from elsewhere in the children's bedrooms. The research confirmed that kids living on farms had lower asthma rates yet were exposed to a wider range of bacteria and fungi than children who did not live on farms.

Importantly, the researchers found evidence that specific types of microbes (found mainly on farms) played a greater role in protection against allergies and asthma.

This was not the first time a study had suggested bacteria and microbes might have a protective role against asthma. In an October 2007 study in *Respirology*, researchers from the *University of Alberta* showed that children under 12 years of age living on farms had a two year incidence of asthma of 2.3 per cent, compared to their rural peers at 5.3 per cent and their urban peers at 5.7 per cent.

"Farm children of ages one to five years also showed a stronger protective effect against asthma than those aged six to 11 years, possibly due to earlier exposure to the farm environment," said William Midodzi, lead researcher on the study.

The Alberta researchers suggested that exposure to endotoxins stimulates the body's immune system and keeps it busy fighting bacteria. They also concluded that, *"This research suggests that we should discourage childhood exposure to tobacco smoke, encourage breast feeding, and not worry about keeping a children's environment too sterile"*.

Other researchers have shown that the small children don't have to live on a farm to develop the immune benefits. A household simply with pets goes a long way towards creating the right environment.

For example, in December 2013, researchers from Michigan University *(Proceedings of the National Academy of Sciences)* exposed mice to dog dust, in a controlled study. The mice exposed to the dog dust (and thus the microbes in it) had much lower inflammation in their airways and produced less mucus than the mice exposed to dust from non-dog households. One microbe in particular, called *Lactobacillus johnsonii*, was very prominent in the guts of the mice exposed to dog-related dust. When the researchers gave a live form of these bacteria to the mice that had not been exposed to dog dust, an equivalent protection against allergens was observed.

Researchers concluded that the results could lead to future studies on how manipulating gut bacteria (by using probiotics or other microbial strategies) might treat or protect children from asthma and other allergies.

Lactobacillus johnsonii may well not be the only relevant bacterium. A research study *(Allergy. 2013 Mar; 68(3):322-9. doi: 10.1111/all.12094. Epub 2013*

Feb 10) looking into farm dust, identified *Staphylococcus sciuri W620* as another microbe that could afford protection against allergic inflammation in airways. There may well be more important strains.

Another study by German researchers *(Journal of Allergy and Clinical Immunology; April 23, 2012)* showed that exposure to bacteria and microbes on cow farms and from raw cows' milk and straw could account for at least half the protective farm benefit. Protection was not just afforded for asthma, but for hay fever, wheezing and eczema. Commenting on the research, Dr. James Gern, a childhood allergy researcher at the University of Wisconsin School of Medicine in Madison, who wasn't involved in the study said, *"Nature can really teach us something here; exposure to non-pathogenic microbes seems to be an important part of the education of the immune system."*

You need to eat a little bit of dirt when you're young. It does you good.

CHAPTER 2
ACTION AND REACTION

There is a simple Newtonian law of physics that states, '*Action and reaction are equal and opposite*'. Something like this is going on here. When a 'foreign' (new to you and your defences) bacterium enters your body a reaction occurs, bacteria are life forms and like all life forms try to make the very best of their living conditions, part of this is that they wish to grow and multiply without being attacked by your body's immune system and so they have developed various ways to protect themselves. For example, one of their defences is to form a 'biofilm' surface around themselves.

If they then can multiply and become numerous enough, the human body will experience their presence as an infection, reacting by building various aspects of the immune defence with new white cells specifically tailored to fight each individual new foe. With each infection, depending upon the severity, you will have a similar reaction – the production of white defence cells and the ensuing fight may well increase your temperature, toxins may be released by the invaders and your body will need to work to neutralise them. You may produce mucus in your airways and a resulting cough. Little Sophie has another 'cold'.

Importantly, your immune system is now 'activated' against this specific bacterium. Specialist, specific antibodies are formed and these trawl your blood and lymph systems. Estimates show that some 85 per cent of your immune system develops in response to these 'foreign' invaders. And even after the fight they may not go away completely. And so your immune system carries specific white cells tailored exactly to fit (and neutralise) each of the 'foreign' microbes for a very long time. As long as some of the microbes remain in and around your body, the defensive antibodies will be present too. And these various tailored defender cells add up to a formidable defensive force. They are your immune memory.

Unlike vaccines, where dead cells may be injected into your blood stream in order to cause this 'reaction' and thus boost the immune system, most microbes involved in natural 'infections' are in your gut. They also tend to endure. Furthermore, a core group 'tops you up' every day; on your food, on your hands and in the air you breathe. Vaccines, on the other hand, may need boosters every few years. And, frankly, you do not know what animal host was used to make those vaccines. Why is this important? As you will see, the immune reaction to an invader is one thing. But the introduction of foreign genetic material into your body is something of major importance.

Obviously, bacteria and microbes come in all shapes and strengths. They are very 'individual' organisms.

Some bacteria are common and relatively harmless, while others can be fatal. The relatively harmless common ones have lived in and around us for millennia and cause an enduring reaction, giving us greater protection when a much nastier and rarer microbe comes along. Of course, you may not have antibodies available that are specifically tailored to the next attacker, but you may have something very similar and thus you have a head start and will be more protected than the next person who does not have the initial protection.

CHAPTER 3

THE SUPER-ORGANISM

It's a fact of life that you come into contact with bacteria throughout every day and night of your life, on your food, on your pillow, in the air you breathe, from your interaction with other people and animals and so on. Bacteria were the first living organisms on this earth over four billion years ago. Today, there are quite probably 5 million different types of bacteria in the world. It is nonsense to think that somehow we could ever stop or even restrict human exposure. But Government Health Authorities, ever fearful of the few dangerous microbes, insist on trying, with misguided and even dangerous consequences.

Ironically, we use bacteria frequently. We don't just coexist with them - we have learned to use them to our advantage. Those on grape skins make our wine, others make certain cheeses and yogurts; some manage our sewage plants or compost heaps for us.

Many food forms helped our 'action and reaction' system by topping us up with the mild, or beneficial, bacteria. Traditional foods like sauerkraut, hung pheasants, blue cheese, raw milk, olives, miso soup and so on, depending upon where you lived in the world.

But governments and health authorities believe that we need to be protected from bacteria. So, certain foods are banned, others irradiated, pasteurised or sterilised.

One hundred and fifty years ago in Western Europe, over 70 per cent of the population was rural; now more than 70 per cent is urban. 92 per cent of the population of America lives in seven per cent of the country. We are no longer brought up on farms breathing the straw and cow dust. In towns we have fewer dogs.

This sanitised world fails us, especially during the first five years of our lives.

Moments before birth, a baby is almost sterile. Babies born by natural birth pick up their first 'infection' when passing through the mother's birth canal. Babies born via Caesarean's do not; they are known to have weaker immune systems and more early illness. They have to play 'catch up'.

Interestingly, research now indicates that the colony of bacteria in the birth canal can play an important role in baby's immune system development. While a healthy mother provides *Bifidobacteria* in her birth canal, a stressed mother can provide less helpful bacteria. Worse, mothers with infections can provide early harmful bacteria. There is a little evidence that one consequence may even be some cases of autism.

What is interesting is that these *Bifidobacteria* are the normal early immunity providers. Although you may have heard a lot about these bacteria, they are not in the top 50 most common bacteria in adult bodies. They are, what's called, Lactic Acid Bacteria (LABs) and apart from enhancing immunity, they also change the acidity in the gut and stop some of the nastier bacteria 'thriving'.

Their numbers are important – they need to overwhelm the opposition. And that's where breast feeding comes in. Breast milk is specifically designed by nature to feed *Bifidobacteria* and thus increase their numbers.

The short-term benefits are clear for a new born baby. But the long-term benefits are starting to emerge too.

2014 research from Northwestern University *(Proceedings of the Royal Society B)* has shown that adults who as a baby were only breast-fed for a limited period, or not at all, have a greater long-term risk of heart problems.

Apparently, there is a correlation between breast-feeding and C-reactive protein (CRP) in the blood later in life. CRP is a predictor of chronic inflammation in the body and the higher your CRP figure, the greater your risk of heart problems.

Babies who were breast-fed for 3-12 months result in adults who have CRP levels 20-30% lower than those not breast fed at all.

Babies take in bacteria and microbes from their very first breath; from the moment you lay them on a pillow and when Dad gives them a kiss.

In our natural environments the mild 'beneficial' (or commensal) bacteria visited us constantly, topping up our stores and thus our immune systems. We lived with them as one. Many of them found a nice dark, damp environment in our intestines with food a plenty. In return they stimulated our immune system and, as you will see, helped us in many other ways. It was a symbiotic relationship, fine-tuned and honed over millions of years.

But we didn't understand this relationship. Many people still do not, even today, doctors and oncologists included.

Yet, in the last decade or so research has been plentiful with over 7,000 studies and several hundred clinical trials. America has already completed a huge $173 million project called The Human Microbiome Project, funded by the National Institutes of Health and involving over 200 top scientists. Now, Europe has the MetaHIT project, often working with the Chinese, focusing on what is called metagenomics. The rush of research started in 2002 and 2003, with 774 citations for published research articles and 77 clinical trials in only a twelve-month period!

The fact is that we need these beneficial bacteria to survive. They are ESSENTIAL TO OUR GOOD HEALTH. I wrote my first article about beneficial bacteria, your friends, your little helpers, in 2005. A Marketing Director from Yakult rang the office saying it was one of the best articles they had read, and I did a second article with their European Head of microbiology on colorectal cancer and its links to microbes. That was nearly nine years ago. How is it that the great majority of doctors and oncologists don't know much about the crucial role of gut bacteria even today? Perhaps it's another 'inconvenient truth' - their drugs don't help the microbiome; they make matters worse, as we will see.

It is a feature of modern science that text book theories consider the human body to be an organism of some seven trillion cells and 25,000 genes. We focus on this organ or that tissue, this knee joint or that breast cancer lump. Our doctors are ever exploring spare part surgery.

But, in reality, we are much more than the sum of the parts. This textbook picture underestimates us. The latest research is very, very clear - the knowledgeable few now regard us as a SUPER-ORGANISM of 100 trillion cells and 100,000 genes, all working in harmony - **a vast, intercommunicating, clever, adaptive, all-providing ecosystem.**

The bacteria on your skin, in your gut, in your mouth and, for females, in your vagina, out-number your body cells ten to one! They provide three times more genes than you have yourself. Think of it! Three times more genetic material directing traffic in your body than your own! Right now! Those genes are constantly making proteins and other bioactive compounds, good and bad. They direct your hormones and even your DNA. They alter the acidity of your gut determining which chemical reactions perform well and thrive; and which slow down and even stop.

Many compounds they make are compounds you simply cannot make yourself. Some can be super-helpful; others can cause chronic inflammation or are pathogenic. Added together, the cells of the microbiome represent the biggest organ in your body, producing more enzymes than even your liver.

Over the millions of years of evolution, we have come to co-exist with the best, the most helpful, the most mutually-rewarding bacteria. Not surprisingly, many of the compounds made by these bacteria are absolutely essential to your growth, development, health and longevity. What happens if they stop making them? What happens if your friendly bacteria become upset?

Their potential to change your life is immense. Welcome to the microbiome.

CHAPTER 4

NATURAL PROBIOTICS AND PREBIOTICS

Say the word 'probiotics' to most doctors and they will think of little milky drinks with more than an added hint of marketing. Write the word 'prebiotics' and they may well think you simply can't spell. So let's clear up a few things:

Probiotic

A Probiotic is most commonly defined nowadays as a supplement containing live microorganisms having a **deliverable** and **proven** benefit in the body. Note the words 'deliverable' and 'proven'. A supplement cannot be called a probiotic unless it has met these two criteria in research.

One of the biggest issues is delivery. Getting the live bacteria through an acid stomach to the point in the intestine where they can deliver their benefit is problematic. This is why beneficial bacteria are often found in small milky drinks or live yogurts, which can afford some protection as the bacteria make their journey.

Lactobacillus casei shirota and *Lactobacillus casei immunitas* are examples of strains of bacteria that meet both criteria of proven delivery and benefit, whereas (and this is why you should be careful) *Lactobacillus acidophilus* is the name of a common species used to make many yogurts. This species has some strains that may meet the probiotic criteria but others that don't. A yogurt 'with acidophilus' is not a probiotic yoghurt unless it says it is on the pot. Many acidophilus strains never reach the large intestine. Saying it contains acidophilus is no guarantee that it is a probiotic. To labour the point: It's not a probiotic if it doesn't say 'Probiotic' on the pot!

Collins Dictionary (Life Sciences and Applied Biochemistry) describes probiotics as 'harmless bacteria, which help protect the body from harmful bacteria'. (Latin: Biota, meaning 'for life'; pro-biotics are thus 'for life').

A wider definition would be that probiotics are any live microorganisms, which are beneficial to human health. Their role was originally suggested in 1907 by Elie Metchnikoff, a Russian Scientist at the Pasteur Institute, who observed that Bulgarians who consumed fermented milk products, with their lactic acid bacteria, lived longer than those who did not.

Certain foods (especially fermented ones) naturally contain probiotics. For example:

- Unpasteurised **Sauerkraut** contains the probiotics leuconostoc, pediococcus, lactobacillus and others.

- **Miso soup** in Japan, popular for breakfast, centres around a fermented soya bean paste. It contains more than 160 bacterial strains.

- **Tempeh** is a fermented soya bean food from Indonesia with similar benefits.

- **Kefir** is a fermented milk product made from kefir 'grains' (a bacteria and 'grain' mix).

- **Kombucha** is a fermented drink of sweetened black tea.

- **Sourdough** bread can contain several probiotics including *Lactobacillus*.

- **Raw milk** contains a variety of probiotics. And several research studies have concluded that raw milk consumption reduces allergies and asthma in consumers.

  * The PARSIFAL study researchers concluded that children who drink 'farm milk' are less likely to suffer from asthma and rhinoconjunctivitis, a condition that causes a stuffed, runny, itchy nose, post-nasal drip, and red, itchy eyes.

  * The *Study of Asthma and Allergy* in Shropshire UK found a lower incidence of asthma among children who frequently drank raw milk. Those who drank raw milk were seventy percent less likely to test positive for allergies to animal dander, grasses, or mites using a skin prick test. They also had on average sixty per cent less total IgE in their blood, which is the type of antibody that contributes to allergic reactions.

  * The extensive GABRIELA study found that

asthma and allergies were inversely associated with raw farm milk consumption but not boiled farm milk.

The investigators of the GABRIELA study visited the farms and took milk samples. Compared to its boiled counterpart, raw farm milk was higher in total bacteria, lactoferrin, IgG antibodies, whey proteins, and TGF-2, which is known to suppress the inappropriate immune responses that underlie autoimmune and allergic conditions.

* A study that surveyed almost 1,000 children living in Crete found that among those without any exposure to farms, those who drank raw milk were about 70 percent less likely to test positive for allergies to cats, grass, mites, or olive blossoms using a skin prick test.

* A study of 320 adults living in Northern Germany found that among the two-thirds of the participants who did not visit farms in early life, those who had been drinking raw milk at the age of six years were 43 percent less likely to have IgE antibodies in their blood against pollen, animal dander, and mites. Among the third who did visit farms early in life, those who drank raw milk were 65 percent less likely to test positive for these allergies.

It should be noted here that a European Study presented in the journal *Food Control*, was concerned that 2-6 per cent of illnesses were caused by consuming milk products and people had to balance the probiotic benefits of raw milk with possible pathogen content (such as campylobacter, salmonella and human pathogenic verocytotoxin-producing *Escherichia coli*).

Other Probiotic benefits

The Mayo Clinic on their website talk of 'encouraging evidence' that probiotics can

- Treat diarrhoea, in adults and children
- Prevent and treat vaginal yeast infections and urinary tract infections
- Treat irritable bowel syndrome (IBS)
- Reduce bladder cancer recurrence
- Speed treatment of certain intestinal infections
- Prevent and treat eczema in children
- Prevent or reduce the severity of colds and flu

Actually, by the end of this little book you will see that they do far more than even that!

Prebiotic

A **Prebiotic** is a food that these beneficial bacteria specifically feed on, which stimulates and encourages their growth and thus the numbers of them that exist in the colony.

The classic example of this is mother's breast milk, which encourages the growth of *Bifidobacterium* in babies, as we mentioned in the previous chapter. The American Academy of Paediatricians notes on its website that:

- Apart from protein, carbohydrate and fat, breast milk provides 'antibodies, immune factors, enzymes, and white blood cells. These substances protect your baby against a wide variety of diseases and infections not only while he is breastfeeding but in some cases long after he has weaned.

- Human milk encourages the growth of healthy bacteria in the intestinal tract of the breastfed baby. It does this by promoting a generally healthy environment and, in part, through substances called prebiotics, which are found in human milk.

- Since human milk stimulates the growth of these 'friendly' strains of bacteria, other bacteria such as *E. coli*, which are more likely to cause disease, are inhibited from growing, multiplying, and attaching to the lining of the intestine, where they can cause infection'.

The website states that babies that are breast-fed (rather than those using Infant Formula milk products) are less likely to develop allergies, wheezing and skin rashes and eczema (even in families with a history of these problems) early in life. Breast-feeding for over six months reduces risks of child lymphoma and leukaemia and is linked to a 36 – 50 per cent reduction in 'sudden infant death syndrome'. There is research evidence too for decreased levels of colitis, Crohn's disease and Type-2 diabetes.

The breast milk doesn't just provide cytokines and antibodies. It contains colostrum and certain sugars like galactose. When these are fermented in the babies' gut by lactic acid bacteria, greater numbers of bifidobacteria thrive and two things occur:

i) More LABs mean more Lactic Acid reducing the pH (increasing the acidity) of the gut further, and thus,

ii) Gram-negative bacteria (the dangerous ones) find it much harder to survive.

Thus, natural birth provides baby with large numbers of *Bifidobacteria* from the birth canal; and, breast feeding specifically increases their numbers and creates an environment in the gut hostile to pathogens. Caesarian birth and bottle feeding babies cannot replicate this.

An American Government overview comments thus:

'The bacterial colonization of the infant gut is a gradual process that exerts a strong influence on the health status, since the members of the gut microbiota may contribute to the barrier effect against pathogens and/or to the maturation of the intestinal immune system. Traditionally, it has been considered that aerobic bacterial groups, such as streptococci, staphylococci, enterococci, lactobacilli, or enterobacteria, together with some strictly anaerobic ones, especially bifidobacteria, are among the first colonizers in breast-fed infants. In concert, they create the condition required for the proliferation of anaerobic bacteria, which become predominant after weaning. In contrast, the microbiota of formula-fed infants seems to be more diverse and prone to changes and contains higher counts of *Bacteroides, Clostridium,* and *Enterobacteriaceae.*

Research on human milk has revealed that this biological fluid is a source of live staphylococci, streptococci, lactic acid bacteria, and enterobacteria for the infant gut. Bifidobacterial DNA has also been detected in breast milk. Bifidobacteria represent one of the most important bacterial groups in the infant gut. In this location, they may contribute to the maturation of the gut barrier and the gut-associated lymphoid tissue. Some studies have suggested that infants with delayed bifidobacterial colonization and/or decreased bifidobacterial numbers may be more susceptible to a variety of gastrointestinal or allergic conditions and that, in these cases, the exogenous administration of selected bifidobacterial strains, alone or in combination with lactic acid bacteria, can reduce the incidence of such conditions.'
(http://www.ncbi.nlm.nih.gov/pmc/articles/PMC2643565/)

Prebiotic foods

So, apart from mothers' milk what are these? Typically they are **whole foods containing indigestible fibre.** For example, fruits and plants contain pectins, which are polysaccharides the body cannot break down or absorb. Pectin is a soluble dietary fibre which binds to cholesterol in the gut and slows glucose absorption by 'trapping' it.

Whole grains like oats, nuts, seeds, greens, vegetables and fruit are good fibre-providing prebiotics, with some, like artichokes, celery, onions, garlic, chicory, bananas, wheatgrass, chlorella, dried fruits, olive oil, aloe vera and Manuka honey shown in research to be especially helpful foods.

But the effect of the prebiotic seems to be specific to the particular bacterium strain and research on this is in its infancy. Some research has taken place: for example, *bifidobacteria* love inulin from onions and chicory, not just galactose from mother's breast milk. Dr John Ellerman, a microbiologist and scientist, who lead a CSIRO research team in Australia of over 120 scientists working on gut flora and health for eight years, is very clear on this. He says that certain strains of *Acidophilus*, for example, are encouraged by specific prebiotics, while other prebiotics can hinder. He has designed a specific LAB Probiotic (*Acidophilus* and *Bifidobacteria*) and Prebiotic mix called *Lactoflora*. Ingesting just a few billion with the right prebiotics can produce several trillion in the gut within 24 hours; more than enough to overwhelm most harmful bacteria with their effects.

CHAPTER 5
MEDICAL MYTHS
AND YOUR IMMUNE SYSTEM

I read a report in the Times where an oncologist was criticising NICE who had turned down a new cancer drug for use in the UK on the grounds that it was not value for money. *'Without the new drug, we will have to keep using Interferon and that doesn't work very well at all'*, was his quote in the newspaper. Interferon and Interleukin are drugs that stimulate an immune response to help the body fight cancer. And, it's true; they are not star performers.

Possibly, it is because simply stimulating the quantity of white immune cells is not enough to be effective. As we have already seen, the immune response has to be tailored specifically to the foreign invader. And this takes time.

In the large intestine (normally, there are relatively few bacteria in the small intestine) the 'good' bacteria have a major role to play. If the good guys dominate, their presence, the acidity of the environment they create, some of the compounds they produce, make it very hard for the invader to progress. However, if a doctor is involved and he has given you drugs, which weaken the presence of the good guys, can they still be expected to act as your strong first line of defence? Can they deliver their normal ability to stop the invader, or at least slow down its progression while your body's immune response kicks into gear?

Of course, there are other factors that are known to impact on your immune system naturally, such as age, hormonal status, and diet. Others, such as laughter, exercise, a good sex life and stress are all indirect factors affecting the hormone system, which in turn affects the microbiome.

Some people are actually known to have a genetic predisposition to bacterial infections *(Hill, 2000)*, although this is rare. For the vast majority of people living without bacterial challenges is attainable.

It is not the purpose of this book to repeat sections of my others (like *'The Rainbow Diet'*, and, *'Everything you need to know to help you beat cancer'*). Suffice it here to say that your immune system is exactly that - a system. When nurses come back to you after a blood test and tell you about the level of your 'white blood cell count', it is virtually meaningless. Your immune system has a variety of different participants each designed to do a different job as part of a complex and highly effective machine. One overall score on your 'white cells' means nothing. You could be missing a vital component. For example, you need a working thymus gland, you need each and all of dendritic cells, B-lymphocytes, T-lymphocytes, macrophages and Natural Killer cells; over twenty members in all.

Next, people read something in their daily paper, pop off down the high street and buy some cheap vitamin pill to 'strengthen their immune system' ahead of the 'flu season'. It is unlikely to help for a number of reasons.

Natural vitamin E helps boost the immune system. In nature it has eight components - four tocopherols and four tocotrienols. The EU in its wisdom will only let you buy a one component version, alpha-tocopherol, and even then it is usually synthetic. The approved supplement is, at best, a copy of a deficient compound - it is a huge over-claim to even call it vitamin E. Nuts, seeds and whole grains, plus certain fruits like apricots are a better alternative.

Vitamin A boosts the immune system, but you should not take supplements as too much can damage your liver. Instead take the pre-cursor beta-carotene. In nature, carotenoids have many properties, immune boosting being one. But beta-carotene naturally occurs in two forms (cis- and trans-). Again the common, cheap high street version is deficient and has only one. Worse, this form should not be used by smokers as it is then linked to an increased risk of lung cancer. Carotenoids are abundant in colourful foods: red and yellow peppers, sweet potatoes, peaches, apricots, greens. As a supplement you might take chlorella, which has good natural levels of beta-carotene.

Vitamin C is regularly quoted as being essential to your immune system. Supplements are often synthetic, and only about seven per cent is absorbed into the body. You can try expensive liposomal versions, which have an absorption of over 85 per cent. But you should be able to eat more than you need on a regular basis. Red peppers naturally contain higher levels than oranges. Try limes squeezed into hot water with grated ginger. Fresh berries are a great source.

Minerals are important too. Both selenium and zinc help these immune boosters to work.

The VITAL study in America showed that the strongest 'common' supplement was grape seed extract; it recorded a score of 46 per cent above the next supplement. It is an OPC. Pine bark extract was not included in the research. It is another OPC and arguably even stronger.

Then there are herbs. Good immune system boosters include herbs such as turmeric (curcumin), cat's claw, echinacea and astragalus. Some of these herbs like curcumin and echinacea involve their polysaccharide content in the way they act. Nobel prizes have been won for explaining how polysaccharides help communications between cells, such as those between foreign or rogue cells and those of the immune system. Some of these herbs plus others like slippery elm bark and liquorice, feed the bacteria too, increasing their numbers.

But.

The diversity of white cells demands a diversity of stimuli. Popping one high street vitamin pill, or a drug like Interferon is unlikely to work across the whole range of white cells. Eating a wide range of foods and herbs, while taking bioactive natural supplements, is far more likely to deliver.

Yet there is another important step. Research over the last few years shows that even if you employ a range of immune system boosters to encourage the full diversity of immune cells to form, this is still unlikely to succeed, without 'activation'.

After boosting the numbers of T-cells and tailoring their structure to the 'foreign' invader, when they leave the lymph nodes to mount their attack, T-cells first need to be 'activated'; and to do this they look for a molecule of vitamin D. Somehow, and it is not fully understood, vitamin K helps in this activation process.

Almost the only natural way to have sufficient vitamin D in your body is through the action of sunshine on the cholesterol stores under your skin. Of course, ridiculous campaigns telling people not to go in the sun and to 'slip, slop, slap', wear hats and stay covered up, have misled people into fearing the sun. A disease caused by a lack of vitamin D, Ricketts, has reappeared in children in the Western world as a result. New obsessions and particularly scaremongering over cholesterol, in part driven by manufacturers of statins, will also dampen people's vitamin D production.

One week lying on a beach in the sun will provide you with 70,000 International Units (IUs) of vitamin D.

Harvard Medical School has recommended 5,000 IUs a day - Professor Holick even stated that there would be 25 per cent less deaths from breast cancer if women had adequate levels of this vitamin in their bodies.

Laughter, a good sex life, exercise, being the correct weight and more are all linked to a stronger immune system. Stress, depression, lack of sleep/disturbed sleep are all linked to weakened immune systems.

Much of this directly involves your hormones. Stress hormones like cortisol can cause chronic inflammation in the body leading to cancer, blocked arteries, arthritis and diabetes. Exercise and sleep can keep this inflammation in check, through hormones like endorphins and melatonin. If inflammation runs unchecked, your immune system is depleted trying to cope with it.

Infection, of course, can have the same side-tracking effect. About 20 per cent of all cancers are 'caused' by infections - parasites, viruses, and bacteria. For example, Hepatitis B and C are linked to liver cancer, *Human Papilloma Virus* to cervical cancer, Epstein-Barr virus to some lymphomas. Viruses and bacteria can drain the immune system, drain the body of certain essential vitamins, whilst producing toxins, some of which are carcinogenic.

This takes us full circle.

A worrying aspect is the frequent comment from oncologists who tell patients to refrain from taking supplements as these might interfere with their chemotherapy. This argument is exposed as nonsense in my book *'Everything you need to know to help you beat cancer'*. Newer drugs are not 'chemotherapy'; major cancer centres like MD Anderson in Texas have conducted research showing that certain drugs are actually helped by certain supplements; and the new breed of bioactive supplements are not the basic vitamin E of yesteryear but curcumin, resveratrol, indole 3 carbinol and vitamin D each of which has a great number of research studies to support it's use in treatments. Curcumin is actually the most researched medical compound bar none, vitamins and drugs included.

Many doctors then tell their patients that they would prefer them to eat 5 lots of fruit and vegetables a day, presumably believing that these could not possibly contain vitamins and natural compounds that might interfere with their wonderful drugs. Bizarrely, most doctors completely omit to tell patients that certain foods conflict with many drugs. For example, eggs and dried meats can conflict with some chemotherapy drugs; grapefruit and its juice can conflict with over 45 drugs involved in all manner of disease treatment! We placed the latest list on the CANCERactive website!

But, as you will see in Chapter 7, telling people to eat their vitamins is actually grossly ignorant, if the medical team has had the patient taking drugs and especially antibiotics. It is not your greens and grains that give you immune boosting vitamin K and B group. It is the bacteria in your gut. They synthesise the vitamins from the raw materials. Without the gut bacteria, you will be devoid of these essential health vitamins and crucial anti-inflammatory compounds like sodium butyrate, which has even been shown to kill cancer cells.

It's just medical mythology at its worst.

CHAPTER 6

THE GOOD, THE BAD AND THE UGLY

The ugly?

Of course not all bacterial infections are mild, harmless and helpful. About 4,000 bacteria have been identified and named by scientists across the world. And these include some that are highly dangerous, for example those causing botulism, typhus and cholera.

The most common bacterial infections across the world include upper respiratory tract and throat infections (from bacteria such as Streptococci), infections in the ear (e.g. *S. pneumoniae*), TB (e.g. *mycobacterium tuberculosis*), then *salmonella, campylobacter, listeria, Helicobacter pylori* and *shigella* in gut and stomach infections.

Other bacterial infections can occur via the skin - impetigo, boils, carbuncles, cellulitis, and complications after cuts and burns (e.g. involving *Staphylococcus aureus, streptococci,* and *pseudomonas aeruginosa*).

Listeria is a dangerous disease. However, researchers at the *Institut Pasteur* in Paris have shown that a healthy microbiome weakens the effects of the foodborne pathogen *Listeria monocytogenes*, restricting its ability to take hold of proceedings in the gut. Pascale Cossart and her team have shown that bacteria in the gut actually programme the host's DNA and RNA to manufacture certain proteins. When a pathogen arrives, the new attacker re-programmes the host protein manufacturing system. But Cossart's research with mice has shown that the stronger the host microbiome, the less the pathogen can multiply, and the less it is able to re-programme protein production (*American Society for Microbiology, mBio, 2014*).

MRSA is a deadly and drug resistant staphylococcus infection, which had the hospital world in a panic in 2010. It is resistant to antibiotics like penicillin and cephalosporins and is a significant problem in hospitals, care homes and prisons. Weakened immune systems coupled with operations, open wounds, catheters and respiratory issues are cause for concern and the disease can grow rapidly in 24-48 hours. After 72 hours it can become serious if not stopped. Several studies have reported that hand washing was a way of limiting the spread of the disease. Restricting the prescription of certain antibiotics is another. The CDC in America found that there were 4.5 cases per 100 hospital admissions. About 3,000 deaths per year in UK hospitals were recorded in 2005. Suggested treatments have included Russian bacteriophages (viruses that attack bacteria), Manuka Honey, the psychedelic mushroom *Psilocybe semilanceata*, cannabinoids CBD and CBG, allicin (a compound found in garlic) and a new composite drug dressing (hydrogen peroxide, tobramycin, chlorhexidine digluconate, chlorhexidine gluconate, levofloxacin, and silver).

But, research confirms the good can triumph over the bad!

MRSA may seem a bad, in-hospital plague to some but another bacterial infection is actually about 25 per cent more common in hospitals and is equally worrying or worse.

Clostridium difficile, or C. *difficile* is a bacterium found in about a third of all children and some 3 per cent of adults. Fortunately, it seems to be kept in check by other bacteria in your body and causes no problems in healthy people.

However, in patients treated in hospitals using drugs and particularly antibiotics, the balance of bacteria in the gut is disturbed and C. *difficile* multiplies, producing toxins, which cause nausea, cramping and diarrhoea. While there is an antibiotic to treat C. *difficile*, it lays waste to all bacteria in the body, even the good ones you need, and doesn't always work, especially in the severe cases.

A decade ago a more virulent strain emerged that can attack individuals after just one routine course of antibiotics. Cases have tripled since that time. This new strain produces up to 23 times more of the disease's primary toxins than the common version.

Like most strains of *C. difficile*, it also produces heat resistant spores that can persist and lead to relapse.

The need for a better treatment is great and urgent. Up to 20 percent of infected patients suffer at least one recurrence; 35 percent of those go on to have a second; and 65 percent of those are likely to have even more. A few sufferers actually have their infected colon removed in order to "cure" the disease.

In 2012, there were over 500,000 cases of excessive *C. difficile* infection in patients treated in hospitals for non-related illnesses in America and 14,000 deaths. The bacterium spreads very easily.

In the 1980s, an Australian doctor, Thomas Borody, suggested that one way to cure patients might be a faecal transplant. (Sorry, I should have warned people who were reading and eating!) The idea is something vets working on farms have known about for a long time. There was even reference to treating humans in America as long ago as 1958. The goal is to restore the ideal natural balance of intestinal flora and over-power the *C. difficile* bad boys.

In 2008, a double blind clinical trial commenced. One of the trial designers was Colleen Kelly, a gastroenterologist in Providence, Rhode Island. She first treated a patient with a faecal transplant in 2008. The patient was completely debilitated after six painful months of *C. difficile* colitis. "*I tried every standard regimen of treatment. Nothing worked*", Kelly says. After the patient received a transplant of her live-in boyfriend's stool, she was completely cured. Kelly had done more than 100 treatments by the start of the trial. According to the *New England Journal of Medicine*, the trial was a success with transplants convincingly beating the best antibiotic for returning patients to health. Indeed, the drugs clearly made matters worse in this trial.

In total, 43 patients were treated. 13 out of the 17 receiving the transplant saw their illness disappear immediately, compared with only four out of 13 in the antibiotic-only group, and three out of 13 in the antibiotic plus transplant group.

As always with these 'natural beats drugs' results, some 'experts' immediately talk about developing expensive pills (which will have to be approved by the FDA as drugs) instead of using the research results and simple enemas. First, you take healthy stools, remove the food and the waste and then give people just the active bacteria in a pill form. The pill is 'guaranteed' to reach its destination and work. *University of Calgary* researchers reported a 100 percent success rate – none of the 27 patients who took the tablet-sized pills had a recurrence of *C. difficile*, even though all of them previously had had at least four bouts of the infection. Patients ingested between 24 and 34 capsules containing faecal bacteria, often donated by family members. *"Patients with C. difficile often have 20 or more stools a day, which seriously affects quality of life and so they are very open to this treatment,"* said Ravi Kamepalli, MD, an infectious diseases physician at the Regional Infectious Disease-Infusion Center, Lima, Ohio, and lead author of the study. *"Human beings are 90 percent bacteria and once that balance is altered with antibiotics, opportunistic infections can cause serious problems. All we are doing with this treatment is resetting the balance."*

The interesting thing will be to see how widespread the use of this pill treatment becomes. While it has been developed to treat *C. difficile*, it could be the corrective factor that might be crucial in illnesses from cancer to autism. How will the treatment be used? Over what time scale? Will it be widely available in hospitals? How much will the 'Super pill' cost? Is this 'super-probiotic' the wake up call to doctors and oncologists in the Western world? Will they now start to understand the damage their drugs cause? Or will its presence make them more 'gung ho'? After all, when a cancer patient goes for surgery and chemotherapy it is now fully understood that their immune system is decimated. Indeed, many illnesses are treated with antibiotics or drugs that damage the microbiome. All traditional surgery comes with lashings of antibiotics.

Maybe all patients should be given this 'super-probiotic' as part of their after care?

One slight complication is the view of The University of Michigan researchers from their on-going Host Microbiome Initiative (HMI) Project that not all healthy people's microbiomes are even consistent, let alone identical. Rather *'each person harbours a unique and varied collection of bacteria that's a result of life history as well as their interactions with the environment, diet and medication use'.*

We shall see.

The Bad?

What we observe above is that you can rebalance your gut by the addition of a full and diverse range of the gut flora from a healthy body. That's the good news. Could it work in reverse? Unfortunately, yes. In research from the University of Michigan using mice, samples of the microbiome community were taken from mice with colon cancer and transferred to healthy mice. These then developed colon cancer at twice the normal rate. Researchers stated that they were *'convinced that it is the community that is driving tumorigenesis. It's not just the microbiome, it's not just inflammation. It's both'* (November 2013 mBio online).

This of course has quite staggering implications, not least could you 'catch' cancer? But the real revelation is that sick bacteria can make you ill.

It was a crucial question, which comes first? Do you develop cancer and this negatively affects your gut bacteria, or do they get sick first? Chicken or egg?

Associate Professor Patrick Schloss PhD, one of the lead researchers, is convinced that sickness in the microbiome bacteria is the driver. In the mice with colon cancer, bacteria such as *Bacteroides, Odoribacter*, and *Akkermansia* were at high levels, while there were lowered levels of the *Prevotellaceae* and *Porphyromonadaceae* families.

But three weeks after the healthy mice had been 'contaminated', they too had similar levels of these bacteria in their gut, and then the colon cancers started to appear. Schloss concluded that the inflammation changed the community and the new community induced the inflammation. *"They make each other worse to the point that you have higher rates of tumour formation."*

Moving on, there seem to be clear links between the bacteria in your mouth and heart disease. In 2010 researchers from the University of Bristol and the Royal College of Surgeons in Dublin showed that tooth plaque and gum disease were a result of Streptococcus bacteria which can build up in the mouth. With gum disease comes the potential for bleeding gums and these bacteria can enter the blood stream. Once there, the bacteria have a protein, PadA, which lines their bodies and this attracts blood platelets, which then clump around the bacteria to protect them from the host immune system. These structures result in clots; they can block arteries, form growths and even heighten lesions in the artery walls and cause inflammation. According to the American Academy of Periodontology, people with periodontal disease are almost twice as likely to have coronary heart disease. A further study – the INVEST study by

Columbia's Mailman School of Health, studied 11 different gum bacteria and found that the heart disease risk pertained whatever the conditions of other factors such as smoking, diabetes and cholesterol levels.

The Michigan University HMI Project referred to above, showed that bacteria can be grouped into 'community types' and those in the mouth were predictive of the community in the gut. *"What was unexpected in our research was that it was possible to predict the type of community a person had in their gastrointestinal track based on the community in their mouth,"* said Schloss.

The Human Microbiome Project in the USA was a five-year study and looked at the colonies of bacteria in 18 different body locations. One conclusion was that the make up of one community is predictive of all the communities. Another was that the bacteria within a community clearly communicate and inter-react.

The researchers also found that a limited amount of data could be ascertained from the community types – for example, whether a person was breast-fed was associated with their gut community type, the level of education was associated with vaginal community type, and gender linked to community types.

Moving on again, some gut bacteria seem linked to diabetes. Dr. Ruchi Mathur from the Cedars-Sinai Medical Center led a team, which showed that some slowdown in the movement of food through the gut is good as this allows more absorption of nutrients.

This seems due to methane-producing bacteria called *Methanobreibacter smithii*. However, an excess of these bacteria is linked to people with a higher body mass index (BMI), more body fat and elevated blood sugar levels. These people take more calories from their food and put on more weight over time.

Finally, another microbe known to cause serious problems in humans and animals is the bacterium *Helicobacter pylori*, more usually associated with stomach ulcers and even stomach cancer. However, there are indications that it may lie behind some Alzheimer's disease (AD). A higher incidence of *H. pylori* has been noted several times in cases of AD. 2012 research from the Institut National de la Sante, Bordeaux *(Neurobiol Aging May 33 (5) 1009)* showed that *H. pylori* infection was associated with increased homocysteine levels (a known link to AD), higher cytokine levels (a known marker of inflammation), gastric atrophy and cognitive impairment.

For your information, the herb goldenseal, together with the mineral bismuth has been shown to deal effectively with *H. pylori* infections. And vitamin B-12, B-6 and folate have been shown to reduce homocysteine levels in the body by a team of researchers at Oxford University – these vitamins even contributing to a 90% reduction in brain shrinkage. As we will see later, these B vitamins are normally manufactured in a healthy gut by your microbiome members.

The Good?

Overweight? Blame your gut bacteria!

Professor Patrice Cani and his team at the Catholic University of Louvain in Belgium has shown just one strain of gut bacteria is capable of reversing obesity and preventing diabetes.

The bacterium in question was a single species of the bacteria *Akkermansia muciniphila*. This normally makes up 3-5% of the total microbiome content but falls dramatically in obese people.

In studies with mice fattened up until they were two to three times fatter than the controls, those then fed the bacterium lost about half their excess weight even though their diet had not changed. The bacterium seems to increase the mucus membrane thickness in the gut, reducing absorption levels. The treated mice also produced chemical signals emanating from the gut, altering changes in the way fat was processed elsewhere in the body. Finally, the treated mice had lower levels of insulin resistance, a key symptom of type-2 diabetes.

A more general study from the European MetaHIT Project Showed that obese people have both less total numbers and less diversity of gut bacteria, resulting in 40 per cent fewer gut bacterial genes than in thin people. As in the Louvain study, they were more insulin resistant and showed more inflammation markers, thus indicating a greater risk of diabetes and heart disease. This Pan-European study, coordinated by Professor S. Dusko Ehrlich at the INRA in France's INRA, indicated eight bacterial species as possible weight gain preventers. Importantly, a second related study showed you could re-boot the microbial richness by changing your dietary habits and using a low fat, healthy diet.

Oluf Pederson who coordinated the Danish part of the project said that the findings indicated you could repair your damaged microbiome and that *'Our intestinal bacteria should be considered an organ just like our heart or brain'.*

There are probably about 800 'types' of bacteria in this 'organ'. About 400 have been identified and named.

While there can be billions of any one strain in your gut, their growth and development can be rapid and determined by the foods you provide. Equally, their decline and even death is also determined by what you feed them. Ever wondered why people told you to eat whole foods and not junk? Now you know. It's not just about nourishing your body. It's about nourishing your friends too. *'You are what you eat'* should perhaps be re-phrased to become *'You are what your microbiome eats'.*

You may assume that leaders of 'the good' bacteria would be Acidophilus and Bifidobacteria and that these are plentiful in the gut, since they are ever present as probiotics on TV and health store and supermarket shelves. You'd be wrong. While people may think that Acidophilus and Bifidobacteria are important gut bacteria, they are not in the top 60 most frequent by volume *(Qin J et al. A human gut microbial gene catalogue established by metagenomic sequencing.* Nature. *2010 Mar 4;464 (7285):59-65).*

Bacteroides spp. are the most common 'commensal' bacteria, with *Bacteroides uniformis* on its own providing almost 10 per cent of all bacterial numbers and therefore genes in the gut. Next come

Alistipes putridinis

Parabateroides merdae

Dorea longicatena

Ruminococcus bromii L2-63

Bacteroides caccae

Clostridium sp. SS2-1

Bacteroides thetaiotaomicron VPI-5482

Eubacterium hallii

Ruminococcus torques L2-14

I doubt you have seen those on a small milky drink bottle in your supermarket!

Different bacteria have very different characteristics and abilities; so bacteria from the general *Lactobacillus* and *Bifidobacterium* offer benefits very different to those of *Escherichia, Enterococcus, Bacillus,* or *Saccharomyces* (a yeast), for example.

Lactobacillus and *Bifidobacterium* are anaerobic

bacteria that produce lactic acid as a result of metabolising carbohydrates. These LABs produce acid themselves and have an increased tolerance to acid, which helps them compete with other bacteria and microbes during fermentation. They are ubiquitous inhabitants of the gut, vagina and mouth.

Strains of Lactic Acid bacteria are the most common microbes employed in fermented foods (sauerkraut, yogurts, olives, pickles) as they inhibit food spoilage. They are the most common constituents of probiotic brands.

The reason why LABs are so common in probiotic brands is that their acid generation changes the pH (acidity) of the gut and quickly holds most of the 'bad' guys in check, restricting their ability to generate toxins or inflammatory proteins and thus stopping potential immune response.

LABs are thus a 'quick fix' - short-term controllers, buying you time to re-introduce the diversity of commensal bacteria back into your microbiome.

It is often thus stated that they are anti-inflammatory. Clearly, the more you have, the better. However, it is not helpful to swallow more than about 10 billion a day. In fact, large quantities can make you sick. Far better to consume a consistent two or three billion three times a day with meals that are high in relevant prebiotic, fibrous foods. Then you will produce the trillions in your gut – more than enough to do the job required.

People who eat a lot of chicory, onions, garlic and leeks tend to have more LABs.

Believe it or not but there is some serious 2014 research into the anti-inflammatory benefits of consuming dark chocolate. Researcher Maria Moore speaking at the 247th National Meeting & Exposition of the American Chemical Society (ACS) explained that LABs (particularly *bifidobacteria*) love cocoa and feed vigorously on it, producing large quantities of heart protecting, anti-inflammatory chemicals.

Clearly such LAB probiotics can make a big difference: Children with diseases such as eczema, allergies and asthma have lowered levels of *lactobacilli*, but an almost adult-like range of *bifidobacteria* species. *(Ouwehand et al 2002)*. This can be addressed through supplementation by the correct bacteria and then a changed diet.

Conversely, consuming antibiotics can make a disastrous difference. In 2003 in Cancer Watch, our research centre, we covered research showing that children who took antibiotics in the first year of their lives had a considerably higher risk of allergy by the age of seven. We also know why. Adaptive immune responses developed and initiated in the mucosal system, especially in the intestine, are essential for healthy immune system maturation *(Rautava et al 2004)*. Local bacterial presence helps develop cytokines *(Romagnani 2000)* and helps build strong infant immune systems *(Holt and Jones 2000)*. Kill these off with antibiotics and the young child is in danger.

We will cover more on antibiotics as we go. Suffice it here to say that it is too easy to think of antibiotics being the medicines from doctors. About 80% of total antibiotic volume in America is destined for animals and fish that are then consumed by humans.

Topping up

Clearly then, good bacteria perform a crucial function, and they need to be present in the broadest spectrum possible, at good levels and so that they dominate and can control harmful bacteria producing pathogens and causing inflammation. While LABs are great in the short-term, the commensal bacteria your body may ultimately need are not necessarily the ones that appear on your supermarket shelves.

But let's start there. You can take your probiotic in a little bottle of fermented milk. Probably the best known is Yakult, which has the potent (and patented) single strain *Lactobacillus casei shirota*. And as you will read, these small drinks certainly have their benefits, but I worry about a sugar content in probiotic drinks of as much as two to three tea spoons a small pot, although there are variants using low fat and low sugar now. Yakult does have some very good supporting research, from modulating the immune response to combating certain infections and relieving constipation.

Multi-strain probiotics can be helpful if they contain five or more strains. For example, Probiota 7, Neways protozymes, Mercola Complete Probiotics can provide a good mix in combination.

It is important you choose a reliable supplier of capsule-based probiotics and, ideally, have the product delivered directly to your home. One Belgian study showed up to 35 per cent of capsule supplements contained dead bacteria and were thus useless.

It is also important not to be lured in by claims of strength. For example, I found claims such as *'Contains 40 billion live bacteria per capsule'* in products in the health shop and on the Internet. 40 billion is too many and, frankly, not how the whole thing works.

The short-term need is LABs; the long-term need is diversity. You need no more than just a few billion **but across a wide range.** The crucial issue is then to **eat relevant high fibre foods to encourage the growth of the most important beneficial bacteria** and the rebalancing exercise.

To demonstrate this point, consider the latest research – for example a study published in *Nature, December 11th 2013.* Researchers took people who ate normal diets and switched them to a high dairy diet of cheese, milk, eggs and meat. **Their microbiomes changed completely in less than 24 hours!** On the animal-protein diet, people showed an increase within their gut in the types of bacteria that can tolerate bile (a fluid produced by the liver that helps break down fat), and a decrease in bacteria called *Firmicutes*, which break down plant carbohydrates. Not surprisingly, the dairy diet saw a greater expression of genes to break down protein, while the plant based diet bacteria expressed genes to help ferment sugars.

The speed of change surprised researchers. Lawrence David, an assistant professor at Duke University's Institute for Genome Sciences and Policy said that *"the choices that people make on relatively short time scales could be affecting the massive bacterial communities that live inside of us"*.

Clearly then, changes to illness patterns might also be made quickly and be diet related.

Diet is crucial in generating a healthy microbiome. But does a diverse diet build diversity in the microbiota? Surprisingly, research is limited. One study with fish showed that eating a more diverse diet did not produce more diversity in the microbiome.

A 2014 research study from Ireland covered in the journal *'Gut'*, looked at sportsmen (in this case, serious rugby players). Despite identical control groups, and both sportsman and the control groups eating a diverse diet, no increase in gut diversity was shown. But when the sportsmen exercised, they increased their gut diversity. The results showed that after exercise the athletes had a significantly wider range of gut bacteria present. One, *Akkermansiaceae*, is known to be linked with lower rates of obesity and associated metabolic disorders. Some people have criticised the research as the sportsmen did eat more protein, but the Irish researchers were adamant that somehow exercise seemed to increase gut bacteria diversity.

The fact is that in the longer-term diversity can only really be regenerated by eating a diet rich in whole, unprocessed foods along with some fermented or even 'untreated' foods like raw milk. Throughout the ages we have consumed foods that had high levels of natural probiotics in them. No longer, as Health Authorities misguidedly 'protect' us from such evils.

Modern diets have also moved away from fibrous whole foods so loved by these important friends of ours. Do you eat an apple a day?

Once you reach the age of 50 the numbers of bacteria in your gut are known to decline anyway. You produce less acid, making it easier for the bad guys to come out to play.

If you cannot eat foods containing natural commensal bacteria then a daily top up is essential with estimates suggesting about 8 billion being the shortfall needing to be replaced each day.

When you take your supplements, do so with cold liquids and a little food. Help the bacteria navigate their way to their goal. Hot foods and drinks will hinder them.

Interestingly, LAB's love of pectins makes apples an important food for increasing their numbers. *'An apple a day keeps the doctor away'* is thus very likely to be true!

Eating protective natural foods

Eating red meat is known to cause inflammation in the body, as does eating fried foods. So fried beef might seem a toxic combination. Certainly researchers trying to fuel metastases in rats thought so. However, imagine their surprise when some of the animals eating this 'bad food' actually recovered from their cancer.

It seems the average cow can be fed many 'unnatural' foods, from grains to even sheep skeletons (this led to CJD outbreaks in the UK, some years ago).

But cows are ruminants – they have rumens where their food mixes with enzymes and commensal bacteria. Fed inappropriate foods, red meat can contain linoleic acid, itself a potential carcinogen.

But the rumen is where grass is normally digested. And grass-fed animals with their natural bacteria instead produce up to 30 different isomers of linoleic acid. These are, it transpires, potent cancer-fighters. Commonly these isomers are called Conjugated Linoleic Acid or CLA *(http://www.canceractive.com/cancer-active-page-link.aspx?n=3551)*.

CLA has been shown to decrease skin, colon, liver and breast cancer, for example, in a vast number of studies and at quite small doses. CLA has even been shown to be taken up by the breast tissue and is both preventative and corrective.

Yet again, nature proves protective.

CHAPTER 7
SO, WHAT ELSE DO THESE HARMLESS BACTERIA DO?

Quite a lot actually.

Firstly, as we have covered, they seem able to direct your immune system and immune memory.

Secondly, depending upon the foods you eat, they seem capable of influencing the acidity/alkalinity of your digestive tract and thus control the success or failure of all manner of chemical reactions.

Thirdly, when the 'good' thrive, they can overwhelm 'bad' bacteria in your body. It's a question of balance, and survival of the strongest.

But there is more; far more:

1. They synthesise unique compounds using their own DNA and RNA. For example, enzymes and proteins that can directly affect your hormones, your nervous system, your immune system and influence and redirect your own DNA and RNA expression. They can also affect the gut lining mucosal membrane and control which compounds attach to important receptors or cross the membrane.

2. They synthesise essential compounds you cannot make for yourself like vitamins and anti-inflammatory agents. For example:

• **Vitamin K**: This is an essential, lipid-soluble vitamin that plays a vital role in the production of coagulation proteins. It is 'found' in green, leafy vegetables and in oils, such as soybean, cottonseed, canola, and olive oils.

K-2 (menaquinone) is, in fact, synthesised by the intestinal flora or colonic bacteria. It is now known to play a protective role against liver disease and metastases to the liver, and it is necessary to the activation of your immune system by vitamin D. You have limited reserves in your body of about one week maximum. *(Medscape: http://emedicine.medscape.com/article/126354-overview)*

• **B Vitamins** like folic acid (essential for correct DNA replication), riboflavin, biotin, and cobalmin (B-12) are produced by Lactic Acid Bacteria. *(Le Blanc et al, Curr Opin Biotechnol. 2013 Apr;24(2):160-8. doi: 10.1016/j.copbio.2012.08.005).* B vitamins have been shown to reduce serum homocysteine levels which seem to pre-stage both cancer and dementia.

• **Sodium butyrate** is synthesised by gut bacteria and plays an important role in reducing inflammation in the body; and also in cell proliferation. It has even been linked with reduced colon cancer risk in African Americans.

Sodium butyrate can turn down an enzyme called COX-2, which causes inflammation in all manner of cells from those in your arteries to those in your colon. Chronic inflammation is known to be a precursor to many chronic illnesses, like cancer, arthritis, diabetes, Alzheimer's and artery damage, strokes and heart disease. For example, chronic inflammation in cardiac arteries allows fat to 'stick' to them resulting in serious heart problems *(Hassan Brin et al; PLOS ONE SLC 5A8 gene transport of butyrate; June 2008, Pubmed)*. In cancer, a gene controlling regular cell division is silenced. Sodium butyrate has been shown to influence the cellular receptor GPR109A to turn the silenced gene back on *(the American College of Georgia, 2009)*.

• **Short chain fatty acids (SFCA)**. Sodium butyrate is not the only short chain ester produced by the gut flora. Others, like acetates and proprionates, produced by *Bacteroides thetaiotaomicron* and synthesized from pectins, help to control and limit the production of LDL ('bad') cholesterol in the body. *(e.g. Gerard Dongowski et al; American Society for Microbiology)*

Japanese researchers from the Riken Center for Integrative Medical Sciences in Kanagawa have shown that gut bacteria producing butyrate from dietary fibre are absent in patients with inflammatory bowel disease. Their studies showed that the reason butyrate was able to reduce inflammation was because it acted as an energy source for cells lining the colon. Without the fatty acid, the gut lining cells made a 'naïve' T-cell, which caused inflammation. When the mice were fed butyrate this converted to healthy T-cells, which stopped the inflammation. The researchers proposed that people with IBS, Crohn's and auto-immune diseases should be given supplements of sodium butyrate with their diets.

Another study, this time from Emory University and published in the EMBO Journal, studied the effects of bacteria from the genus *Lactobacillus* on the epithelial lining cells of the gut. Looking across a number of animals, they showed that the animals with the bacterium in their guts produced Reactive Oxygen Species (ROS), which then stimulated production of new stem cells and this produced a healthier gut lining. In particular, *Lactobacillus rhamnosus* was particularly helpful in healing where the gut lining had been damaged by exposure to chemicals and microbes. *"Unlike most cell types that cannot tolerate bacterial contact, intestinal epithelial cells respond to Lactobacillus rhamnosus by increasing their motility"*, said lead researcher Andrew Neish.

3. They can bind to, and eliminate, dangerous compounds you would rather not have in your body. Heavy metals like cadmium and mercury; and nitrosamines and oestrogenic products (both chemical and human) can be eliminated by chelation – binding to bacteria working with fibrous foods like lignans and pectins.

Modified citrus pectins, biodegradable biopolymers and sulphur and methyl compounds produced by gut flora, using a variety of fibrous foods including plant chelators, have been shown to be a part of the process in removal of dangerous toxins from the body.

Some bacteria can even feed on pesticides and eliminate them from the body:

One research study looked at the role of microorganisms in the degradation of the organophosphorus insecticide chlorpyrifos during kimchi fermentation.

During the fermentation of kimchi, the insecticide degraded rapidly until day 3, and had degraded completely by day 9. Four Lactic Acid Bacteria were identified as being responsible for the effect.

According to the study, as reported by Green Med Info:

"(The bacteria) were identified as Leuconostoc mesenteroides WCP907, Lactobacillus brevis WCP902, Lactobacillus plantarum WCP931, and Lactobacillus sakei WCP904. (The insecticide) could be utilized by these four strains as the sole source of carbon and phosphorus."

Dr. Natasha Campbell-McBride is a Russian medical doctor with two Masters degrees, one in Nutrition, the other in Neurology. One of her special subjects is gut bacteria. On her website she comments *"The digestive track all spread out would cover a tennis court, and it is the perfect place for anything harmful in the environment to settle. Yet the good bacteria there chelate chemicals and toxic metals – if they can't destroy it, they grab it and take it from the body.*

In one research study, two groups of rats were given organic mercury. One group were given a powerful antibiotic, the other group were not. The mercury got into the blood stream of only about 1% of those without the antibiotic, but 90% of those with the antibiotic. Keep gut flora healthy and strong and it will protect you. Healthy gut flora will chelate mercury and remove it from the body".

4. A healthy microbiome can prevent a myriad of diseases: As we saw in the last chapter it is almost certain that your microbiota becomes ill or out of balance first; and their imbalance is linked directly with a wide variety of illnesses.

Campbell-McBride has a full-time medical practice in the UK where she treats children and adults suffering from autism, learning disabilities, neurological disorders, psychiatric disorders, immune disorders, and digestive problems. She has developed a theory on Gut and Psychology Syndrome (GAPS), which, in her opinion, can make a child particularly prone to vaccine damage. Her GAPS Nutritional programme is designed to treat illnesses naturally, such as autism, ADHD, dyslexia, dyspraxia, schizophrenia and depression.

Her view is that nearly every disease – both physical and psychological - originates in the gut. She is not alone in that view. Her conclusion is that once you heal and seal your gut lining, you start to heal the disease. She is not alone in these views:

a) In *Nature: 488, 178–184; 9 August 2012,* Marcus Claesson and a team of about fifteen experts reported that alterations in intestinal microbiota composition were associated with several chronic conditions, from obesity to inflammatory diseases.

b) In 2007 Frank, D. N. et al. linked the make up of the microbial community imbalances directly to human inflammatory bowel diseases *(Proc. Natl Acad. Sci. USA 104, 13780–13785; 2007)*.

c) A study in 2012: *(Jeffery, I. B. et al; Gut 61, 997– 1006; 2012)* linked IBS directly with species-specific alterations in faecal microbiota.

d) Chronic inflammation is linked to all manner of illness like cancer, heart disease, diabetes, rheumatism, arthritis, and obesity. Gut flora thus play a crucial role *(Ley, R.E, Turnbaugh, P. J, Klein, S. & Gordon. J, Nature 444 1022-3; 2006)*.

e) Ageing is also directly linked to flora composition and the microbiota of older people displays greater inter-individual variation than that of younger adults. In research on 178 elderly subjects, analysis of faecal matter showed correlation with residential location, illness and rehabilitation. The microbiota composition correlated with diet and age, but also with illness and frailty. Flora composition declined with age-related frailty.

According to *Science* magazine *(6 June 2012)*, **the human gut microbiome contributes 36 per cent of all the small molecules that are found in human blood,** passing such molecules across the gut wall, and it '*plays a major role in creating susceptibility to certain human diseases*'.

'*In recent years, a variety of microbial communities have been characterized through such efforts as the Human Microbiome Project and the Earth Microbiome Project. But mapping these trillions upon trillions of microbes and analyzing the vast amounts of data that are accumulating will require new integrative approaches aimed at understanding how microorganisms function and are interrelated*'.

Both *Nature* and *Science* argued that your microbiome actually becomes 'ill' first, just as Campbell-McBride above and The University of Michigan researchers found. It doesn't like the toxins and poisons you don't like. And, until it recovers, you cannot. So, it would seem the new 'super-probiotic' may be an essential 'drug' for all manner of illnesses.

The American Gut Project

University of Colorado researchers, amongst others, are organisers of the American Gut Project, in association with the Human Food Project, and are recruiting thousands of people to donate their gut bacteria to science. It is also cross-related to location. Anyone in the world can participate. The project follows on from the Human Microbiome Project (the $173 million NIH-funded project I mentioned earlier). *(See http://americangut.org/)*

A donation of $99 will have your gut bacteria examined, and compared with your dietary record. It might tell you crucial things about what you have in your gut.

To quote from the website, *"While researchers are cautious and right not to oversell the microbiome (much work is still needed to confirm causation for many ailments), the direct or indirect implication of microbes in a staggering number of ailments and diseases of the modern world, reinforces that* **we are on the cusp of a paradigm shift from the orthodox notions of health and disease"**.

Personally, I think this shift is going to happen very quickly. I think the numbers of scientists involved, the growth of 'genetics' as a science in American Medical Schools, and the realisation that the genes in the microbiome can control your health is an unstoppable force. You will see research coming thick and fast in 2014 and 2015. And that research will put a very big question mark over drugs. They may even one day be moved to 'Treatments of last resort'.

CHAPTER 8
THE FIRST LINE
OF DEFENCE

The bacteria in your gut perform another important function. They are your foot soldiers – your first line of defence against the yeasts and microbes that entered your body with your daily food and drink. Whilst your commensal bacteria love whole, fibrous foods, they adore certain microbes, fungi and yeasts, particularly yeasts like *Candida albicans*.

At night, while you sleep, if the right conditions of acidity/alkalinity exist and the beneficial bacteria are plentiful enough, they will consume over two pounds by weight of yeasts, fungi and microbes. Yummy!

If they are unable to do this, the yeasts and microbes in your body will eventually prevail. The toxins they may produce, along with their very presence, alters the pH of the fluid inside the gut, making it less acidic and more favourable to their existence. Thus their colonies will grow and as the acidity levels decline further (i.e. the pH increases). They will increasingly and detrimentally affect the essential biochemical reactions in your gut.

So the result is a 'double whammy': More bad guys and thus more toxins, inflammation and even an 'auto' immune response; plus, a lowered production of crucial messages that positively affect your health.

Yeasts can cause holes in the gut lining. This damage is also termed 'leaky gut syndrome' and yeasts escape into the blood stream. There they can colonise small areas of the body and, as they are anaerobes, they may starve those areas of oxygen. This can have dire consequences. Chronic illness and even cancer is a possibility. One research study in 2007 concluded that women who had taken 25 or more courses of antibiotics in their life times, had double the risk of breast cancer. Antibiotics will severely damage the levels of beneficial bacteria in the gut flora, allowing an over expression of yeasts.

Yeasts may also stick to receptor sites on cell membranes preventing the cell from receiving important messages. Research, also in 2007, showed that the use of cinnamon could reduce the symptoms of type-2 diabetes by 25 per cent. Cinnamon is known to kill yeasts in the blood stream. It would seem that eradicating them may, in some instances, allow the insulin receptor sites to work more efficiently.

The late Gerald Green wrote articles for CANCERactive and was an expert in gut health, often advising hospitals on patient strategies. In his article *'Can candida cause cancer?'* he firmly believed the title possible. He advocated a sugar-free diet with neither glucose (including refined carbohydrates) nor cows' dairy (and its sugars like lactose).

He explained that a diet involving sugar or after-meal fruits and soft vegetables like marrows or courgettes could promote fermentation by the yeasts, where upon, the patient would suffer bloating, fatigue and even feel 'hung over'. Women might experience thrush and cystitis; men might have yellow toenails and flatulence. Beer and alcohol would also similarly encourage the growth of yeasts at the expense of the good bacteria.

While many people focus on yeast dominance and its links to IBS, colitis, and Crohn's, yeast infections cause much more havoc throughout the body. For example, they may be a serious threat to life in some cases of leukaemia where stem cell treatment has taken place. They themselves can cause chronic inflammation and a leaky gut can allow quite large molecules into the blood stream resulting in increased levels of illness. A greater explanation is provided by the National Candida Centre on their website, *'Candida overgrowth can lead to 'leaky gut syndrome', which is medically referred to as 'intestinal permeability'. Leaky gut is a major gastrointestinal disorder that occurs when openings develop in the gut wall. These tiny holes can be created when candida overgrowth moves to a more serious stage and the candida yeast grows roots or hypha, the long, branching filamentous cell of a fungus.*

The hyphae spread the bowel wall cells apart so that acidic, harmful microorganisms and macromolecules are then able to leak through these openings and enter the circulatory system.

Leaky gut syndrome and candida infection can

directly lead to many other systemic inflammatory and immune-related symptoms beyond food allergies, such as rheumatoid arthritis, ankylosing spondylitis, multiple sclerosis, eczema, fibromyalgia, Crohn's disease, Raynaud's phenomenon, chronic urticaria (hives), and inflammatory bowel disease'

But there's another issue. The overgrowth of bacteria in the small intestine, which normally contains very few bacteria compared to the large intestine. Intestinal permeability coupled with an overgrowth of certain bacteria in the small intestine has been shown to cause non-alcoholic fatty liver disease, or NAFLD. Italian researchers looked into gut permeability in patients with NAFLD and compared the results to patients with untreated coeliac disease, who are known to be prone to this condition, and to healthy volunteers. Interestingly, they concluded that while bacteria overgrowth and/or permeability were causal, probiotics could relieve liver problems caused by a high fat diet.

As with yeast infections, bacterial overgrowth in the small intestine is associated with bloating, constipation or diarrhoea, leaking gut, fatigue, depression, headaches, asthma and food intolerances; just to mention a few symptoms! As I suggested above, one main food to avoid is glucose (and foods and drinks containing it), which not only feeds such infections, but causes much gas production, and toxic waste products.

Natural Yeast killers

Gerald Green's anti-yeast diet focused on starving the

yeasts of the sugar they crave whether it be common glucose and refined carbohydrates or sugars like lactose in cows' dairy. His was primarily a grilled fish and meat diet with a lot of steamed vegetables and salads. But there are herbs and bioactive compounds that can help. The Chinese herb wormwood is particularly effective against yeasts, as are pau d'arco, natural oregano, cinnamon, caprylic acid, garlic and chillis. Another effective treatment for intestinal yeasts is a teaspoon of sodium bicarbonate in warm water.

Microbial parasites may need a little more. An effective treatment, involving a variety of herbs like cloves, slippery elm and black walnut, is a product called Parafree, from the company Neways (Modere). Wormwood *(Artemesia vulgaris)* again helps here, and a combination of the herb goldenseal and bismuth are effective against the bacterium *Helicobacter pylori*, as I mentioned earlier.

Govindsamy Vediyappan, assistant professor of biology at Kansas State University and his team have shown that *Gymnema slyvestre*, a tropical vine plant found in India, China and Australia, known for benefits in controlling sugar levels in diabetics, is a potent herbal treatment for *Candida albicans*.

If you do think you have a parasite and you treat it with herbs, remember that your wife, husband, partner may be infected too and you both need treatment or you may just pass the pathogen backwards and forwards between you.

Faecal Transplants

Australian Professor Thomas Brody has been championing faecal transplants for 25 years. His treatment programme includes diseases such as Crohn's, colitis, auto-immune diseases and even neurological diseases. Now two of Australia's top teaching hospitals (St Vincent's in Sydney and Perth) are embarking on a large National trial, such they feel is the potential.

The Australian CSIRO's chief research scientist, David Topping, believes the world is on the point of an enormous health breakthrough. *"I think we're on the edge of something quite extraordinary. The attention has switched entirely to the large bowel bacterial population, which we now know is absolutely critical to human health"*.

Borody is not waiting for the Australian clinical trials. He knows faecal transplants work. He claims to have been using them with great success for years on patients that come from all over the world. He has the testimonials to prove it. For example, Suzanne Heskett, an Australian nurse, seriously ill for 13 years with Crohn's is now cured after using a nasal tube into the small intestine in a five hour 'operation'. Eleven months after the treatment, a colonoscopy showed that she was completely clear. Where a year before she had needed to go to the toilet 18 times a day, she was now living a normal life. Heskett has been completely clear now for 12 years.

Emiterus Professor, Robert Clancy endorses that faecal transplants are safe and 'a game-changer'. *"We are looking at everything afresh"*, he said. *"It makes sense that molecules can get into the body's system and change it, while affecting immunity and causing allergies"*. Topping goes further, *"This holds immense potential for the management and prevention of serious diseases, colorectal cancer, inflammatory bowel disease, perhaps even conditions like Alzheimer's, autism and Parkinson's"*.

CHAPTER 9
THE GUT-BRAIN
CONNECTION

Much work has been done since 2010 on the connection between gut bacteria and the brain. In a review article entitled 'Voices from Within' *(Cell Mol Life Sci. 2013 Jan;70(1):55-69. doi: 10.1007/s00018-012-1028-z. Epub 2012 May 27)*, authors Forsythe and Kunza note the following:

'Bacterial colonization of the intestine is critical to the normal development of many aspects of physiology such as the immune and endocrine systems. It is emerging that the influence of the gut microbiota also extends to modulation of host neural development. Furthermore, the overall balance in composition of the microbiota, together with the influence of pivotal species that induce specific responses, can modulate adult neural function, peripherally and centrally'.

So, it would seem that gut bacteria play a role in brain and nervous system development and also in common mental and 'mood' processes. Certainly psychologists are becoming very interested.

One study - a colloaboration between the Karolinska Institute in Sweden and the Genome Institute in Singapore in 2011 - looked at the effect of gut bacteria on brain development in mice *(PNAS)*.

The research team compared behavioural patterns and gene expression in two groups of mice. One group were raised from birth with normal microbiomes, while the others were kept bacteria-free (germ-free). By the time they had reached adulthood they had completely different behavioural patterns and the researchers concluded that their respective brains had developed differently.

The adult bacteria-free mice were observed to be more active/energetic and engaged in more adventurous and 'risky' behavior.

Where the bacteria-free mice were given bacteria when young, they too developed 'normally'. But when only given the bacteria as adults there was no change in their 'risky' personalities.

The researchers went on to profile the genes of the respective mice and assessed signaling pathways involved in learning, memory and motor control.

"The data suggests that there is a critical period early in life when gut microorganisms affect the brain and change the behavior in later life," commented Dr. Rochellys Diaz Heijtz, lead researcher.

Professor Sven Pettersson, coordinator of the study, added that not only were signaling chemicals like serotonin and dopamine subject to regulation by gut bacteria, synapse function also appeared to be regulated by them too.

The implications, of course go well beyond the growth of mice into adulthood; the colonisation by bacteria in evolution has developed and/or limited our brain power too.

The Forsythe and Kunza review also noted that *'There is now robust evidence that gut bacteria influence the enteric nervous system, (ENS), an effect that may contribute to signaling to the brain. The vagus nerve has also emerged as an important means of communicating signals from gut bacteria to the Central Nervous System.'*

Indeed, a bidirectional link between mental state and the gut is nothing new. Experiencing sadness or stress is known to affect the gut; imbalances and infections in the gut can cause mood swings in return.

Teams of researchers at America's top Universities are studying the connection between your gut bacteria and your brain and specifically how they affect mood swings, attitudes and diseases from Autism to Alzheimer's. For example, at UCLA, Professor Emeran Meyer M.D. has been studying the link between the bacteria in your gut and how your brain functions. An analysis of 60 humans showed that different regions of the brain were stimulated as a result of the dominance of different gut bacteria.

Professor Stephen Collins at McMaster University, Ontario, Canada has studied timid mice and fearless mice. And not only do they have different gut bacteria, but when you put the timid mice bacteria into the fearless mice intestines, they too become timid.

Premysl Bercik, an associate professor of

gastroenterology at McMaster University originally observed that a significant number of his patients were not only suffering from gastrointestinal problems, but also from emotional problems such as depression and anxiety.

So in 2010, Bercik and his team studied this and discovered that *'Mild gut inflammation caused by chronic parasitic infection... induces anxiety-like behavior in mice'*.

In 2011 they too researched two types of mice - timid and adventurous mice (Balb/c and NIH Swiss) - and showed that bacteria from one type could change the behavioural patterns of the other *(How the Microbes Living in Your Gut Might Be Making You Anxious or Depressed; AltNet)*.

There is still a great deal to learn but already it is known that bacteria such as *Bifidobacteria dentium* produce an inhibitory neurotransmitter known as GABA, as does a strain of Lactobacillus; while Bacillus and Serratia produce dopamine, a neurotransmitter that activates the reward and pleasure centers of the brain but is depleted in cases of Parkinson's disease.

Other McMaster's team members have been working with University College Cork on which species of bacteria affect the activity of which genes in the brain.

In bacteria-free mice brain-derived neurotrophic factor (BDNF) was significantly up-regulated; this would mean that factors essential for normal brain development would be decreased. Other research showed high levels of serotonin in the hippocampus of bacteria-free mice; serotonin is known to increase stress and cause mood swings.

A third gene (encoding the NR2B subunit of the NMDA receptor) has been found to be down-regulated in the amygdala of bacteria-free mice.

All three genes have previously been implicated in emotion and anxiety-like behaviours.

The subject of Autism can be hugely controversial. In a 2013 meta-analysis of available research *'Gastrointestinal Concerns in Children with Autism: What do we know?'* for the Autism Science Foundation in America, Doctors Barbara McElhanon of Emory School of Medicine and William Sharp of the Marcus Autism Center in Atlanta observed that:

i) There has been a rapid increase in the numbers of cases to 1 in 88 children born (according to the CDC, 2012). This has prompted a level of urgency amongst carers.

ii) There has been frequent reporting of gastro-intestinal symptoms *(Croen et al., 2012)*.

iii) There has been a fivefold increase in reported cases of feeding problems *(Sharp et al., 2013)*.

The results of the meta-analysis suggested children with ASD are at increased risk for gastrointestinal issues[1]. Specifically, greater levels of gastrointestinal symptoms reported by parents compared with siblings (roughly an 8 fold increase in the risk) with areas of specific concern including abdominal pain, constipation, and diarrhoea.

Certainly there is 2012 research showing that kids with autism were twice as likely as children with other types of disorders to have frequent diarrhoea or colitis, an inflammation of the large intestine.

Researchers from Arizona State University's Biodesign Institute have showed that autistic children have different gut bacteria to 'normal' children with one species of gut bacterium completely missing. And these may first enter the baby during transit of the birth canal. It also seems that stressed mothers can have stressed babies and that the relevant bacteria are also passed during the passage through the birth canal.

Research into gut bacteria and autism is actually gathering pace[2].

Clearly it's early days yet but one issue is whether the bacteria are sending chemical signals to the brain and/or are affecting nerves in the gut, which then stimulate the brain. In one study it was noted that 20 genes were affected by a reduction in Lactobacillus levels. And these genes covered the growth of brain nerve connections and even the development and growth of brain cells *(Society for Neuroscience, California)*.

Elsewhere in the book I cover the emerging knowledge of the relationship between bacteria and brain illnesses such as Parkinson's, Alzheimer's and dementia.

Clearly, the idea that microbial or parasitic infection can affect your brain development, your mood swings and ultimately the demise of this organ is massive. The implications concerning the connections with the gut via chemicals and nervous system are so great that the microbiome has even been dubbed the 'second brain'.

Already psychologists are talking about the possible use of faecal transplant treatments to overcome behavioural issues and chronic mood problems in patients. Some of these 'patients' are currently behind locked doors!

The presence of a particular bacterium is also a community issue. Before travel around the globe became so easy, communities were more geographically confined. Scientists can now hypothesise why one race might have been more aggressive while another was more passive.

Skeptics might also contemplate that microbes could be the next weapon in warfare. Let's be quite clear. In the experiments with mice, those who had the highest levels of antibiotics and were 'germ-free (bacteria-free) were the most aggressive.

Certainly, at a simple level, it is easy to see why countries such as Russia are refusing to have GMO foods anywhere inside their borders.

Accidental or deliberate, gut bacteria have the potential to control your mind, your attitudes and your actions, not just your health.

* *

Further references

(1) Buie T, Campbell DB, Fuchs GJ 3rd, Furuta GT, Levy J, Vandewater J, et al. Evaluation, diagnosis, and treatment of gastrointestinal disorders in individuals with ASDs: a consensus report. *Pediatrics.* 2010;125(suppl 1):S1-18

(2) Mulle JG, Sharp WG, Cubells JF. The gut microbiome: a new frontier in autism research. *Curr Psychiatry Rep.* 2013;15(2):337. doi: 10.1007/s11920-012-0337-0. Epub 2013 Feb 15

CHAPTER 10
PLANT
BENEFICIAL BACTERIA

There is another ecosystem involving bacteria that is crucial to your health. Yet again this ecosystem is ignored by health and medical authorities although there are numerous research studies explaining its importance.

Dr Daphne Miller of *Farmacology* believes that it may be the soil where the food is grown, rather than just the food *per se*, that also keeps us healthy.

Living soil to Miller is soil teeming with microorganisms like bacteria, fungi, protozoa, and microscopic roundworms called nematodes. These microorganisms are essential components of life. There is a crucial relationship between the soil's ecosystem and the rhizosphere, the root ball environment that ultimately dictates the nutrient absorption from the soil.

Then we have yet more friends that we have evolved with over the millennia: insects. They eat the bad guys in the soil that might cause us harm. So the rhizosphere is like the gut in humans; it is a bacterial processing system that has evolved to live in harmony with us. Pour pesticides and herbicides on it, destroy the bacteria and fail to replenish the fibrous content and, ultimately, our health must suffer. Leaving a field to lie fallow in the Middle Ages helped to replenish the soil with nitrogen-fixing bacteria, helpful bugs and fibrous material. The subsequent plants then absorbed more 'life' for us to eat. The more ecologically we farm, the more nutrients we harvest.

Plants have proven relationships with each other - through aerial emissions of volatile gasses they emit, and also through the mycelial networks around the root balls in the soil. Children living on farms don't just have microorganisms from cows on their pillows, but microorganisms from healthy soils. Over the millennia, the DNA of such microorganisms has been shown to incorporate into our very own DNA. One research study on sea-dwelling Japanese showed DNA from seaweed incorporated into the gut DNA of the fishermen.

It really is time to sort out your own vegetable patch, to plant some fruit trees and to build a compost heap!

What the implications are for people who consume their expensive salads from Hydroponic farms no one seems to have addressed. The salads, red peppers and herbs are grown in pieces of rock wool, with constantly flowing water under their roots. The water contains 'all the nutrients the plants need' according to the expensive websites. Unsurprisingly, there is no mention of helpful bacteria on these websites.

Weapons of mass destruction

Of course you have to be concerned by modern farming methods. Not just are there less bioactive natural compounds in mass produced food (see the detailed report in *'The Rainbow Diet'*) but governments have no concept of the increasing research into the soil's own microbiome, and its destruction by pesticides and herbicides.

Worse, we are now exposed to largely un-researched, genetically modified foods. If a company like Unilever wants to launch a new food brand, it must go through hoops to have the product approved before it can launch. This is just not true for genetically modified foods. The American Government even told the Food and Drug Administration (FDA) to keep out, leaving companies like Monsanto to 'self-regulate'. It's a scandal.

France is a lone voice in Europe – The Caen Study showed high levels of tumours in animals fed GMO foods, complete with pictures. France wants these unapproved seeds and foods banned from Europe.

Russia has refused to countenance GMO foods inside its borders after tests involving a potato crop produced increased rates of cancer. China has expressed alarm too.

Even the FDA has expressed concerns; not just that genetic modifications may end up in the gut DNA of generations in the future, but that some GMO foods have their own built-in 'bacteria destruction systems'.

The FDA has expressed serious concerns that these same genetic modifications could act against essential 'good' bacteria in the human gut.

The 'game changer' was the incorporation of a gene from the soil bacterium *Bacillus thuringiensis* into crop seed genetics. This gene actually produces an insecticide, *Bt* toxin, which inside the gut of an insect causes the gut lining to fail. *Bt* spores then cross into the blood stream and the insect is no more.

The manufacturers of the GMO seed took the stance that the *Bt* toxin was perfectly safe in humans, but as early as 1999 a study in the Lancet was confirming FDA fears – after just 10 days of consuming GMO feed by rats, their cells and linings of the stomach and intestine showed 'significant' alterations.

As so often is the case, the warnings went unheeded.

But independent research has continued. Research in *Nature* has shown contamination by the *Bt* gene in both pregnant women and their foetuses. Indeed, research has shown that a staggering 80 per cent of new born babies in America test positive for *Bt* in their gut.

Human gut beneficial bacteria *Clostridius* seem to lose ground to the more pathogenic *Enterococcus* bacteria in animals grazing in fields, which had previously contained GMO crops. A 2004 study showed that the gut bacteria had received the *Bt* genetic modifications identical to those given to the GMO soya seed.

This study followed one in 2002 from Newcastle University where the uptake by gut bacteria of *Bt* was measured in people who were healthy, or those who had had their colons surgically removed. Needless to say, the *Bt* toxin passed straight through the no-colon people, but the healthy people had no evidence of *Bt* in their stools – it had all been taken up by their gut bacteria.

A November 26th 2013 report from the Institute of Responsible Technology, using American Government data, talks of five areas of damage in the human gut because of GMO foods:

1) Permeability increases

2) Imbalances in the microbiome

3) Immune system activation

4) Impaired digestion

5) Damage to the intestinal wall

There is also evidence of increased sensitivity to gluten.

If Monsanto and their rivals think GMO seeds are safe, then they need have no fear of any research results. It is puzzling then that despite the outcry, there is still little research and even less transparency.

In May 2009, the American Academy of Environmental Medicine (AAEM) called on, *"Physicians to educate their patients, the medical community, and the public to avoid GM (genetically modified) foods when possible and provide educational materials concerning GM foods and health risks."*

Calling for a moratorium on GM foods, they demanded long-term independent studies, and GM content labeling.

AAEM's clear stance was that, "Animal studies indicate serious health risks associated with GM food including infertility, immune problems, accelerated aging, insulin regulation, and changes in major organs and the gastrointestinal system". AAEM's conclusion? *"There is more than a casual association between GM foods and adverse health effects. There is causation."* as defined by recognised scientific criteria.

More and more doctors in America are already prescribing GM-free diets. Ohio allergist Dr. John Boyles said *"I used to test for soy allergies all the time, but now that soy is genetically engineered, it is so dangerous that I tell people never to eat it."*

Even this is not enough. There's another problem being created by GMO giant Monsanto, via its herbicide, Roundup.

The active ingredient in Roundup is glyphosphate.

The problem comes in two parts:

(1) The direct effect on humans and their gut bacteria. An on going research project and review by Drs Stephanie Seneff and Anthony Samsel at the Massachusetts Institute of Technology argues that Roundup is probably the most harmful toxin humans have ever encountered. The researchers

propose that glyphosphate is the most significant causal factor in today's epidemic of gluten intolerance and coeliac disease in the USA and Europe. The review points to research where fish exposed to glyphosphate exhibit digestive problems and gut bacterial imbalance. It also reviews the effect of glyphosphate in chelating minerals and depleting amino acids – the review identifies lowered levels of certain enzymes, minerals (for example, iron cobalt and copper) and amino acids such as tryptophan, tyrosine and methionine.

(2) The effect on helpful soil bacteria. It has always been argued by Monsanto that Roundup is safe because it targets the shikimate pathway, and this is unique to plants.

Again Seneff and Samsel have shown that glyphosphate affects human CYP proteins. CYP1B1 cytochrome P450 is unique to cancer cells and Professors Potter and Burke in separate experiments believe this gene is your natural protector gene. It takes certain bioactive compounds (they call them pro-drugs) and converts them into new compounds (for example CYP1B1 converts resveratrol into picetannol) and these new compounds kill the cell – the cancer cell – leaving healthy cells, which do not have the gene, unharmed. Glyphosphate seems also to affect the *p53* gene, the controller of normal cell division.

But let's get back to the theme of the chapter – bacteria. **The shikimate pathway is also used by bacteria.**

So, bacteria in the soil are harmed by Roundup. No one apparently even considered this possibility when GMO seeds were launched, even though Monsanto were arguing that the GMO crops were immune to Roundup, so it could be sploshed all over the fields without harming the GMO crops. Monsanto's marketing from the outset claimed Roundup was 'environmentally safe' and biodegradable. 'Untrue' claimed the French and in 2009 a court upheld two earlier convictions against Monsanto for false advertising in France of Roundup.

Glyphospate has a potentially devastating effect on soil bacteria, reducing the presence of the good guys (especially the nitrogen-fixing bacteria), restricting diversity, while allowing immune pathogens to dominate. There is even research showing that somehow Roundup inhibits the uptake of minerals into plants because it interferes with the fulvate system (a chemical that aids the mineral absorption process into the plant).

But, of course, as weeds become immune to Roundup, farmers are encouraged to splosh on even more. So, how much of these sprayed products do you eat? A crucial question because glyphosphate is known to have the potential to affect the shikimate pathway in the commensal bacteria in your gut too!

CHAPTER 11
GUT BACTERIA AND VACCINATION

There's an obvious question in all this. If your gut bacteria trigger your immune system and result in 85 per cent of your immune memory store, how does all this interface with vaccination?

Research in this area is in its infancy. But clearly there is great concern over exactly what is going on, now the importance of gut bacteria in conferring immunity has been established.

The sceptics point to the dangers of introducing foreign DNA and RNA contained in vaccines into your body, and the potential damage of vaccine carriers such as the heavy metal, mercury. Other concerns include the question of what happens to a small baby, whose immune system started as a blank sheet of paper, and instead of developing when passing through mother's birth canal, weaning on mother's milk and slow exposure to new bacteria down on the farm, it is accelerated with a dramatic shot of a potential pathogen, however treated to neutralise it and make it safe. Does a vaccine enhance or threaten the fragility of the baby's developing microbiome?

In a 2011 paper[4] researchers from Canada noted

that clinical trials showed oral vaccines against polio, rotavirus and cholera had less efficacy and blunted immune response with individuals in developing nations; in these cases, they stated, the individuals have greater gut diversity than individuals in the developed world.

A 2012 study[5] looking at whether a rotavirus vaccine had any effect on gut bacteria concluded there was none whatsoever. Vaccinated children had the same gut diversity and numbers as unvaccinated children. However, the vaccine was administered orally, and this is known not to be as effective as systemic vaccination because children in poorer populations have thicker mucosal membranes in their gut.

At a conference in India, Professor Gagandeep Kang confirmed this but went on to also state that systemic vaccinations that worked at a 100 per cent level in Mexico, had fared far worse in India. His hypothesis was that the Indian children became infected with the diarrhoea-causing virus at a much earlier age when either their own gut bacteria were at a much lower level and less able to 'help', or they still had high levels of maternal antibodies which neutralised the vaccine. The conference also heard several speakers talking about increasing the diversity of gut bacteria, and healing leaky gut syndrome, in these poorer children by the use of probiotics. A fair degree of confusion seems to exist! [6]

However, in 2013, three studies[1, 2] resulting from a collaborative effort between the *University of Maryland School of Medicine Institute for Genome Sciences and the Center for Vaccine Development* seemed to offer quite different results.

The first study examined the impact of an oral typhoid vaccination on the gut bacteria; the second looked at the impact of vaccines against Shigella, but this time in monkeys.

A further third study looked into what happens when the gut bacteria are exposed to wild-type Shigella, which as with *S. Typhi*, gain access to the body orally *(PLOS ONE)*.

The first conclusion was that the magnitude of the response depended on the existing diversity of gut bacteria. The more diverse the existing gut bacteria, the greater the resistance to infection by wild type Shigella. No surprises there really.

But the greater the diversity of gut bacteria, the more the characteristics and magnitude of the immune responses to the vaccines was too. *"Our research raises the intriguing possibility that the gut microbiota may play an important role in response to vaccines and susceptibility to enteric pathogens, or bacteria that affect the intestinal tract,"* stated Claire M. Fraser, PhD, professor of the Departments of Medicine and Microbiology and Immunology and director of the Institute for Genome Sciences (IGS) at the University of Maryland School of Medicine.

The first study analysed what happened to the human gut microbiota when an oral typhoid vaccination using *Salmonella Typhi (S. Typhi)* was given. Sure enough, the gut bacteria were affected; and it seems that the more diverse the microbiome members, the stronger the immune responses to the vaccine.

This same conclusion was reached in the test with monkeys and *Shigella dysenteriae 1*. Here the monkeys had been vaccinated, and were then 'attacked' by the pathogen. Where the monkeys had more diversity, the vaccinated monkeys had stronger immune systems. Where they had less diversity, the more the wild bacteria infection took hold. Again, the results don't seem surprising.

What was surprising was that where they had more diversity anyway, the vaccine was less effective. The stronger your immune system, the more it counters the ultimate infection and also the vaccine too.

"This area will continue to be a target for our research as we try to learn more about these pathogens, how they affect the body and how we can prevent infection with these sometimes deadly illnesses," said the lead researcher.

Answers or Problems?

While the researchers above thought this was a major step forward, sceptics merely found the use of vaccines without a full understanding of their impact even more worrying. To put this in context, a child in America, if the Government CDC recommendations are followed to the letter, will receive 49 doses of vaccines in 14 shots by the age of six. By the age of 18 this reaches 69 doses in 16 shots.

Worse, 26 doses by the age of one, is double the dosage rate of countries such as Sweden.

Clearly, from the Maryland research, no two children have exactly the same volume or diversity of gut flora. They may have been born naturally, or by Caesarian; breast fed for a short or long period, or only bottle-fed; they may have received antibiotics, or vaccinations at different levels.

The research itself evidences the fact that vaccination is being mandated by governments and their health departments without a full understanding of exactly what is happening inside the body. The research is being done after the decision, not the other way round – this is hardly rigorous 'evidence-based' medicine!

In a 2001 chickenpox outbreak in Maryland (by coincidence), 75 per cent of the children developing the disease had actually been vaccinated.

Indeed, there is a concern that exposure to vaccines in urban caesarian-born, bottle-fed infants that simply do not have the gut bacteria diversity that children used to have down on the farm is resulting in an INCREASED death rate.

According to the American National Vital Statistics Report, more than 26,000 American babies born alive in 2009 died before their first birthday; about six per 1000.

That figure is higher than in Europe and has seen America actually fall from 12th to 30th in world rankings of infant mortality. All this in the country that provides the most vaccinations. Coincidence or not? Certainly, this is not a well-enough researched area in which to be mandating treatments on the fragile and varied gut microbiomes of babies.

Also, the Maryland vaccine and gut bacteria research only looked at the response differences, not whether there was any effect on the microbiome itself. And this is a big void in our knowledge especially now research shows foreign DNA can be taken up by the gut bacteria, AND, any imbalance in the gut bacteria may produce chemicals that can impact the brain directly via the nervous system and/or through chemicals, or indirectly through an immune response, especially in the young. It is all a little too worrying.

What has been shown in the research covered earlier in this book is that autism is linked to a lowered diversity of gut bacteria. And the Maryland study shows that this will definitely cause a different response to vaccination, than in a child with a much more diverse microbiome community.

Sceptics also point at statistics: in the mid-90s 1 in 10,000 children had autism in America, but by the year 2000 this had increased ten-fold to 1 per 1000. The most recent CDC figures show this as a shocking 1 in 88. Sceptics point at vaccinations – whether it's the vaccine, the DNA/RNA introduced, or the mercury carrier.

But there may be other reasons; and there may be a dozen different forms of autism. No one truthfully knows yet.

What is also known in autism is that a lack of diversity in gut bacteria is coupled with gastro-intestinal problems and the over-presence of some more dangerous inhabitants. As detailed earlier, some 'stressful bacteria' have even been shown to be picked up during passage through mother's birth canal, for example if she has been ill, has an infection or if she herself is stressed.

Ironically in all this, researchers at the University of Guelph in Ontario *(Vaccine, August 2013[3])* think they have developed a vaccine to control at least some of the symptoms of autism, by knocking out the effects of *Clostridium bolteae*, known to worsen some of the properties of autism in children. The vaccine involves yet more bacteria, which target carbohydrate on *C. bolteae's* surface. The research was conducted using rabbits and a human vaccine is likely to be 10 years in preparation. The question someone sensible in authority needs to ask is, *'Is developing a vaccine to counteract one possible symptom the real issue?'* Shouldn't we stand back and analyse what factors might be causing the disease in the first place? Yet again, we see an emphasis on more drugs rather than prevention. Vaccines to 'cure' a problem that vaccines may have caused in the first place? The medical world is dangerously close to spiraling out of control.

So, do strong gut flora and diversity help or hinder vaccines? Do the vaccines enhance or hinder them? And why do poorer populations seemingly have poorer responses to vaccinations, even systemic ones?

Maybe it's another inconvenient truth. Poorer populations who eat more than their fair share of 'dirt' may have more advanced microbiomes. The lowered effectiveness of vaccines may be because the gut bacteria simply regard the vaccine constituents as another rogue attack and deal, pretty effectively, with the intruder – without developing any immune memory. But this begs the question, why don't they actually deal as effectively with the real pathogen when it attacks?

There are many such mysteries still to be solved. Would it not be sensible to hold fire on at least some of the infant vaccinations while some of the more vexing questions are answered? After all, medical science likes to generate this aura of rigour and clinical testing before drugs are introduced into the body. Aren't vaccines, with their DNA/RNA genetic material and as yet unknown actions on the microbiome, just drugs – wolves in sheep's clothing?

* *

References for this chapter:

1. Anna M. Seekatz, Aruna Panda, David A. Rasko, Franklin R. Toapanta, Emiley A. Eloe-Fadrosh, Abdul Q. Khan, Zhenqiu Liu, Steven T. Shipley, 2. Louis J. DeTolla, Marcelo B. Sztein, Claire M. Fraser. Differential Response of the Cynomolgus Macaque Gut Microbiota to Shigella Infection. (PLoS ONE, 2013; 8 (6): e64212 DOI: 10.1371/journal.pone.0064212)

2. Emiley A. Eloe-Fadrosh, Monica A. McArthur, Anna M. Seekatz, Elliott F. Drabek, David A. Rasko, Marcelo B. Sztein, Claire M. Fraser. Impact of Oral Typhoid Vaccination on the Human Gut Microbiota and Correlations with S. Typhi-Specific Immunological Responses. (PLoS ONE, 2013; 8 (4): e62026 DOI: 10.1371/journal.pone.0062026)

3. Prof. Mario Monteiro, University of Guelph, http://www.uoguelph.ca/news/2013/04/guelph_scientis _1.html

4. Rosana B. R. Ferreira, L. Caetano M. Antunes, and B. Brett Finlay, Glenn F. Rall, Editor; PLoS Pathog. 2010 November; 6(11): e1001190. Published online 2010 November

5. García-López R1, Pérez-Brocal V, Diez-Domingo J, Moya A. (Pediatr Infect Dis J. 2012 Dec;31(12):1300-2. doi:10.1097/INF.0b013e318269e3ec)

6. http://www.iavireport.org/Back-Issues/Pages/IAVI-Report-15(6)-AGutResponsetoVaccines.aspx

CHAPTER 12
BREAKING THE DEAL

As I said earlier, beneficial bacteria in our microbiome are our essential long-standing friends. The deal was that we would be a good host, providing a home that was dark, moist, at the right pH, and full of fibrous, whole foods. In turn they would make important vitamins and short chain fatty acids that we needed, while stimulating a strong immune defence, devouring yeasts and microbes, and clearing heavy metals and certain toxins from the body. This symbiotic relationship was a very good deal for us humans.

Unfortunately, we didn't keep to our side of the bargain.

We failed to feed them properly. We don't feed them enough whole fibrous foods like seeds, nuts, olive oils, vegetables, fruits and indigestible fibres like lignans and pectins. Instead we feed them junk: refined carbohydrates, trans fats, glucose-rich fizzy drinks, crisps, beers, pot noodles and worse. They don't like sugar and refined carbohydrates. These foods actually feed their enemies.

We don't top them up like we used to. Our foods are pasteurised, irradiated, treated and boiled. We don't eat 'a bit of dirt' in our modern world. We moved away from the farm. We stopped having pets. We even shampoo our dogs!

We also poison our friendly bacteria! We put chlorine in our water to kill them. We treat our foods with pesticides and herbicides and these linger under the polish of apples, or in the red and orange pigments of certain bright fruits, which you eat and transport to your gut.

We change the acidity of their environment – we consume too much salt, too much alcohol, too many pickles and vinegar; we smoke, we get stressed.

Then we travel to exotic countries or eat their imported fruits and consume new bacteria our friends have never had to deal with before.

It's not just GMO foods that can threaten your essential bacteria – we eat meat laced with antibiotics and the occasional drug. Our tap water in cities is recycled. German research showed it contained drugs, oestrogen (the female sex hormone) from contraceptives and HRT, and even aspartame from sweeteners! These are all new to our friends. Can they deal with them? Who knows?

We also pop pills directly - drugs and antibiotics – with increasing abandon. The attack is indiscriminate. Of course antibiotics don't just destroy the bad guys. They randomly attack the good guys. Some decline 10 per cent, some 50 per cent. And the one you got from touching the dog and putting your fingers in your mouth was completely wiped out. How are you going to replace that one? A three-week treatment with antibiotics is regularly used in animal experiments to clear the whole gut of bacteria. Yet, I regularly speak to people with cancer who have been on five or six weeks, and sometimes more, of antibiotics to eradicate an infection caused by the original medical treatment and which won't go away. Do you really want your gut to become sterile? Especially now after you have read what your friends can do for you, and how sterile guts disrupt your normal mental functions.

Then we wash with triclosan-containing, anti-bacterial soaps and shower gels. We have fluoride and triclosan in our toothpastes. We gargle with strong anti-bacterial mouthwashes. In Cancer Watch we covered research from Perth School of Medicine, which showed an 8-fold increase in throat cancers amongst people who smoked and/or drank alcohol, but also used an alcohol-based mouthwash regularly. *'If it were a face cream, it would be banned immediately after our findings,'* concluded the lead researcher.

What chance do our friends have? What chance do we have without them?

Not surprisingly, these life forms adapt. They are very good at adapting. Some divide every twenty minutes or so. That is a lot of genetic replications, any one of which can produce a new, stronger strain, equipped to withstand our drugs, our antibiotics and our pesticides. And there is no evidence as yet that these new strains will stick to our original deal. We didn't. Why should they?

Right on cue comes a comment from Dr Arjun Srinivasan, a high-ranking official with the Centers for Disease Control and Prevention in the USA. In an interview with Frontline he said this:

"For a long time, there have been newspaper stories and covers of magazines that talked about 'The end of antibiotics, question mark?'"

"Well, now I would say you can change the title to 'The end of antibiotics, period'."

Srinivasan went on to say, *"Both humans and livestock have been overmedicated to such a degree that bacteria are now resistant to antibiotics."*

As you will see in Chapter 14, many illnesses are linked to a reduction in the diversity of bacteria in the gut, often linked to an excess of bacteria that cause chronic inflammation. A whole swathe of 'auto-immune' diseases may well originate in the gut.

But do we learn from this? Do we reconsider GMO foods, the explosion in the use of drugs, the widespread sterilisation of our urban world? We may have to, and very soon.

CHAPTER 13

GUT BACTERIA AND COLON CANCER

A few years ago, I was talking to Britain's top Colon Cancer Charity about causes of colorectal cancer for an article I was writing. Below is a list of factors that they believe increase risk:

Although the charity told me there was a link to coffee consumption, no one could provide the research references. Alcohol consumption can increase risk. Red meat consumption is supposedly causal. Certainly it is linked to inflammation in the body and vegans have lower levels of cancer. Saturated fat consumption causes the production of carcinogenic bile acids such as deoxycholic acid and lithocholic acid each linked to localised inflammation and increased cancer risk. Smoking increases colorectal cancer risk.

The charity also believe you can best prevent colorectal cancer by employing a diet high in fresh vegetables and fruits. From Cancer Watch we know that there is American research that suggests that 3 different parts of the colon may be protected by 3 different vegetable consumption patterns, but the Boston Nurses Study was re-analysed by Harvard Medical School and the only vegetable that seemed to have a significant beneficial link was garlic.

Colon cancer is known to be presaged by localised

inflammation, which causes polyps and these can progress into cancer.

The Japanese develop higher levels of stomach and colon cancer, but then there is a link to smoking, pickles and vinegar (they have a higher consumption of pickled foods), and microbes and parasites typically found in raw fish and sushi.

What else can I add?

The development of colon cancer has been linked to localised oestrogen by both UK (Birmingham) and American Medical Schools (UCLA). Nitrosamines (typically from burned meat in barbeques) can also increase the risk of both colon and stomach cancers.

Colorectal cancer patients are known to have much lower plasma levels of vitamin D, and certain B vitamins like folic acid, biotin and B-12. Vitamin D can reduce risk levels of colorectal cancer and is known to reduce the carcinogenic bile acids mentioned above.

I have long held the view that the way we treat colorectal cancer is flawed. It has long seemed to me that the 'symptoms' (or is it causes?) of colorectal cancer are really properties of an out of control microbiome.

Two close friends have had the disease and in both cases a significant part of their intestine was removed and, whatever the actual words spoken by the surgeon, they both came away thinking they were clear of cancer. This is just false hope at its worst. Colorectal cancer seems to metastasise at a very early stage. Often two years after the initial treatment, secondaries appear in the lungs and sometimes the liver. If it was all cut away, how could this be true?

Obviously, as I always tell people, cancer is a disease of the whole body. In this case it just appeared first in the colon.

My own theory has been simply that the intestine became 'upset'; that the natural flora and the ecosystem were seriously out of balance. And we have known since John Vane won his Nobel prize in the 1990s that this can result in chronic inflammation, and reduce crucial cancer-fighting compound production by our friends.

In 2007, American research carried in Cancer Watch confirmed that colorectal cancer could well be microbial in origin. That fitted my two friends' backgrounds. One almost died when, twelve years before, after attending a wedding reception where hard boiled eggs had been adorned with mayonnaise and left in a very hot tent for 5 hours, *Listeria*, endless drugs and hospitalisation were the result. My other friend had battled yeast infections for years, again by taking prescription drugs.

In both cases, their bacterial ecosystem was clearly badly compromised. Lack of B vitamins? Inflammation? Failure to remove oestrogenic or nitrosamine compounds? Garlic (a well-known microbe controller) the only vegetable that clearly makes a difference? (Although high-fibre diets may well play a part). I talked to a surgeon who told me they often saw yeast growth in the colon of patients.

Research from Leeds Medical School in 2010 showed that the inflammation and polyps could be controlled by concentrated fish oils. But it is also known that small (75mg) doses of aspirin, curcumin, ginger and garlic can reduce the activity of the COX-2 enzyme that is largely responsible for these problems.

So, is there really no opportunity to try to calm the situation, calm the inflammation and rebalance the ecosystem, maybe with the new faecal transplant super-probiotic? It just puzzles me how anyone could think that chopping out a length of your colon could possibly cure you.

Isn't it time to explore a route that at least tries to restore the microbiome to its full glory? So many features of colorectal cancer point in the same direction like changed pH, possible yeasts, previous illness, low blood level of B vitamins, localised oestrogen, inflammation etc.

Different gut bacteria may cause colon cancer

Researchers, part of the extensive SYNCAN study, have now found that people diagnosed with colon cancer have fewer different beneficial bacteria in their gut than healthy people. And those they do have feature more harmful strains (*Journal of the National Cancer Institute, December 2013*).

"*For the first time, we found that colorectal cancer patients have a different gut bacteria composition than healthy subjects,"* said study author Jiyoung Ahn, an assistant professor of epidemiology at the NYU School of Medicine in New York.

Researchers found an increased presence of inflammation-causing *Fusobacterium*, which is also known to fuel the growth of some cancers. Patients also had lowered levels of *Clostridia*, a bacterial class known to aid glucose metabolism.

Researchers also noted that diet, exercise and weight control would alter the composition of the microbiome. All have been linked to lowed risk.

So at last, research on the microbiome is confirming my concerns and theories of the last decade.

Colorectal cancer is caused because the microbiome is greatly disturbed through parasitic infection, loss of diversity and reduction in sheer numbers of commensal bacteria (probably due, somewhere along the line, to drug and antibiotic taking). Factors such as vinegar, alcohol, stress and smoking which will all alter the pH of the gut make matters worse, as does not feeding your friends their favourite high-fibre foods.

All too often, the orthodox treatment of choice for parasitic infections or chronic yeast infections is drugs and antibiotics. How can that help? Surely that will only make matters worse, further reducing the numbers and diversity of the gut bacteria and hurting the crucial participation of the good guys.

Please, let us not keep trying to tell patients their illness is their own fault, when the first action is to put drugs into the patient and chop away a chunk of their colon.

Remember the research I talked of earlier involving mice with colon cancer. Taking the microbiome from mice with colon cancer and giving it to healthy mice brings on colon cancer at double the normal rate in the healthy mice. The bad guys are very powerful. They have to be the subject of the medical response. Cutting out a chunk of colon, prescribing drugs and antibiotics leaves them in the colon and reduces their enemies, the good guys.

Hopefully, sense will now start to prevail as more and more research comes on line.

CHAPTER 14
SICK TO YOUR STOMACH!

This is probably the most important chapter in the book. Here I simply try to show you that research in just the last 18 months confirms what I started telling CANCERactive readers nearly ten years ago. Each research study may seem tiny. But some of the conclusions are huge. And the addition of all these studies together leaves anyone with an open mind in little doubt. The paradigm shift in medicine has started.

In April 2012, The Mayo Clinic and the University of Illinois researchers, while researching Rheumatoid Arthritis, stated that *'The billions of bugs in our guts have a newfound role: regulating the immune system and related autoimmune diseases.'* A healthy microbiome is anyway affected by diet, exercise and hormones, and *'as you age changes occur which further modulate the gut immune system and exacerbate inflammatory conditions in genetically susceptible individuals'*.

"The gut is the largest immune organ in the body," said co-author Bryan White, Ph.D., director of the University of Illinois' Microbiome Program in the Division of Biomedical Sciences and a member of the Institute for Genomic Biology. *"Because it's presented with multiple insults daily through the introduction of*

new bacteria, food sources and foreign antigens, the gut is continually teasing out what's good and bad. The gut has several ways to do this, including the mucosal barrier that prevents organisms — even commensal or 'good' bacteria — from crossing the lumen of the gut into the human body. However, when commensal bacteria breach this barrier, they can trigger autoimmune responses. The body recognizes them as out of place, and in some way this triggers the body to attack itself", he added.

So, the largest immune organ in the body, genes that make vitamins and essential compounds, but also inflammatory chemicals, small molecules that spread throughout your blood stream, auto-immune diseases, illnesses from arthritis to diabetes. This is enormous!

Which illnesses may involve our friends and enemies? Let us have a short look at a little of the very latest research. My recommendation is that you read all that follows, not just the illnesses relevant to you. In that way you will see the important emerging picture very clearly.

First, though, let me start with two extremely common illnesses that affect almost all of us at one time or another:

1. Coughs and colds

Researchers *(King S. et al, Brit Jour Nutrit, April 29, 1-14, 2014)* have conducted a common literature review across eight databases and concluded that adults and children with common respiratory diseases took less time off work or school and were ill for less days, if they were taking a daily probiotic, especially a *Lactobacillus* or *Bifidobacterium* strain.

2. Diarrhoea and/or Constipation.

People who go abroad on holiday and develop diarrhoea understand that they have developed an infection in the gut. The vast majority take some medicine, which kills these 'nasties' and they think no more of it. Of course, the killing field was not confined just to the nasties, and most probably probiotics, especially LABs, would have worked just as well without any collateral damage.

When people develop constipation rarely, if at all, do they think they have developed an infection in the gut. Rather they resort to traditional thinking and eat more fibre, more fruit or drink prune juice. The fact is that removal of fibre from the diet doesn't cause constipation, so why would adding more fibre to the diet help? Indeed, there seems to be an increasing amount of evidence that too much fibre can cause stools to be too bulky and less easily passed.

It is becoming obvious that constipation, like diarrhoea, is caused by gut infection. There certainly is research that shows people with chronic constipation have a different composition of bacteria in their gut than normal. The actual rogue bacteria (it may not be confined to just one) looks to be a type of a clostridium, for example *C. tetuni, C. difficile, C. botulinum* or *C. perfringens*.

The reasoning for this is that constipation sometimes responds to an antibiotic (Vanomycin) known to kill these guys.

In animals born with no gut bacteria, food is passed slowly through the gut. As bacteria levels rise, so food passing reaches more normal rates. As I explained earlier, one area of the gut contains a section of your nervous system (the Enteric Nervous System), which connects to your brain. This system ensures gut movement.

Gut bacteria can influence this nervous system by the chemicals they produce and the Clostridium boys will produce toxins that slow down the whole movement.

There is research, for example some pilot studies, with pregnant women or children. A mixture of probiotic bacteria including various strains of *Bifidiobacterium* and *Lactobacillus* seems to ease constipation rapidly. (The research studies used *Bifidobacterium bifidum* W23, *Bifidobacterium lactis* W52, *Bifidobacterium longum* W108, *Lactobacillus casei* W79, *Lactobacillus plantarum* W62 and *Lactobacillus rhamnosus* W71).

Other studies have investigated the effects of individual strains of probiotics *(Refs 1-7 below)* on the symptoms of constipation with probiotic strains, such as *L. shirota* and the *B. infantis*, increasing defecation frequency and softening stools in adults with constipation. Another with children showed an increase in defecation frequency and a decrease in abdominal pain using the strain *L. rhamnosus.*

When LAB probiotics are provided it results in a lowering of pH in the colon and this enhances peristalsis.

The bottom line (sorry – couldn't resist it) - constipation should be thought of in the same way as diarrhoea. It's an imbalance in your gut flora and both can be 'corrected', at least temporarily, by the use of probiotics.

Now let us turn to some other illnesses:

3. Arthritis

Let us start this section with the illness that was the special subject of my American in Dubai, arthritis. There is arthritis, often occurring after damage to a joint, and there is rheumatoid arthritis (RA), which is known to be strongly influenced by diet.

My friend had RA in both hands. An allergy test linked it to shellfish. He hasn't eaten them in five years and has totally recovered.

RA is a chronic inflammatory disorder that can cause pain, swelling, stiffness, and loss of function in the finger, wrist, and other joints throughout the body. It occurs when the immune system mistakenly attacks the body's own tissue, such as the membranes that line the joints.

Environmental factors, such as cigarette smoking, diet and stress, are thought to play a role in triggering the disease. Historically, treatments have usually involved medications to relieve pain and reduce inflammation. That might well be ending.

The gut microbiome has been linked to arthritis in animal studies. To confirm this in humans, a team of researchers from NYU School of Medicine examined 114 people, some who were healthy, some who had been newly diagnosed and untreated rheumatoid or psoriatic arthritis *(November 5, 2013, eLife online)*.

The researchers found that 75 per cent of people with arthritis had the bacterium *Prevotella copri* in their gut microbiome, whereas it was only present in 21 per cent of the healthy group. Further studies showed it was present in only 12 per cent of already treated RA sufferers and 38 per cent of people with psoriatic arthritis.

However, this may not be the only factor. The heightened levels of *P. copri* linked to reduced levels of other bacteria like *Bacteroides*, known to play a role in reducing inflammation.

Next the research team investigated DNA samples from the bacteria and showed that specific *Prevotella* genes correlated with the presence of RA.

A further study was then performed, this time to see if *P. copri* actually caused inflammation. First the team gave healthy mice a dose of *P. copri*. Then the mice were given a chemical that caused colitis, which inflames the intestine. The ones with *P. copri* had far worse inflammation *(Expansion of intestinal Prevotella copri correlates with enhanced susceptibility to arthritis. Elife. 2013 Nov 5;2(0). pii: e01202. doi: 10.7554/eLife.01202).*

4. Autism

People with Autism tend to suffer more gastro-intestinal problems than the norm. In *Cell, Dec 19th, 2013*, University of Colorado Boulder Professor Rob Knight commented on the first study from a group of American researchers in the newly formed Autism Microbiome Consortium, saying, *"This study strengthens the scientific understanding that what goes on in your gut affects what goes on in your brain"*.

In the study, researchers led by Elaine Hsiao of California Institute of Technology used a development called maternal immune activation to induce autism-like symptoms in mice. Those with this condition had gut microbial activity widely different to the control group of normal mice. When the mice with autism symptoms were fed the bacterium *Bacteriodes fragilis*, the behavioural symptoms were greatly reduced. Researchers found that levels of 4-ethylphenylsulfate were 46 fold heightened in mice with autism-like symptoms but *Bateriodes fragilis* reduced these levels to normal. The researchers also showed that hundreds of other compounds were at changed levels, not just 4-ethylphenylsulfate, which showed the most marked change.

"Scientific evidence is mounting that the trillions of microbes that call the human body home can influence our gut-linked health, affecting our risk of obesity,

diabetes and colon cancer, for example. But more recently, researchers are discovering that gut bacteria can influence neurology – possibly impacting a person's cognition, emotions and mental health" said Knight. Researchers are still not sure exactly how the effects are communicated to the brain. It may be chemicals passing through the body, it may be that those chemicals cause other inflammatory responses, or it may be that the gut bacteria have an effect on nerves in the gut and these communicate with the brain.

This study followed 2012 research by the Centers for Disease Control and Prevention amongst thousands of children with developmental disabilities, which showed that kids with autism were twice as likely as children with other types of disorders to have frequent diarrhoea or colitis, an inflammation of the large intestine.

Another study *(PLOS ONE, July 3rd, 2013)* by Rosa Krajmalnik-Brown and Jin Gyoon of Arizona State's Biodesign Unit. In this study researchers showed that kids with autism had a greatly reduced spectrum of gut bacteria. One in particular, *Prevotella*, was completely missing. Amongst children with autism, GI problems such as pain and constipation can be a real problem but research has suggested that poor levels of gut bacteria may trigger inflammation which reaches the brain. Dr Daniel Smith Senior Director of Discovery Neuroscience said that these studies suggested a need to take a whole body view of autism.

5. Blood Pressure

Researchers from The Johns Hopkins University and Yale University, (11 February 2013 online issue of *Proceedings of the National Academy of Sciences*) have found that gut bacteria maintain the body's normal blood pressure. Apparently a special odour sensing receptor (Olfactory receptor 78) found in the nose, is also present in blood cells, and this senses changes in the gut metabolism. But there is also a non-odour receptor too (Gpr41).

The researchers showed that the controlling factor was the Short Chain Fatty Acids produced by the gut bacteria in a healthy gut. When the SCFAs bind to Olfr78, blood pressure rises; when they bind to Gpr41, it falls. Gpr41 has the stronger effect, so eating a healthy meal has a more positive effect immediately.

In another study, this time by Karlsson FH, Fak F et al *(Nat Commun. 2012;3:1245. doi: 10.1038/ncomms2266.),* the gut bacteria that cause arterial wall inflammation were even identified. Researchers showed the bacteria even modified host metabolism. In patients with atherosclerosis in the carotid artery and linked to cerebral events, especially strokes, the bacteria *Ruminococcus* and *Collinsella* were in high quantities. In the healthy controls, *Roseburia, Bacteroides* and *Eubacterium* were enriched.

Patients with atherosclerosis were also found to have higher levels of bacterial genes making peptido-glycan, were depleted in phytoene dehydrogenase and had lower levels of β-carotene. Healthy people have bacteria that produce more lycopene and β-carotene, two compounds that reduce inflammation. Importantly researchers particularly **emphasised the importance of the changes made by the bacterial genome.**

6. Crohn's and Colitis; IBS

Lesions in the ileum (the small intestine) in Crohn's disease are characterised by *E. Coli* invasion, which actually replicates within the cells lining the gut *(Lapaquette P, Darfeuille-Michaud A. Abnormalities in the Handling of Intracellular Bacteria in Crohn's Disease.* J Clin Gastroenterol. *2010 Jul 7).*

Ordinarily, the number of bacteria is greatest in the large intestine (at least 1,000,000,000 bacteria per millilitre of fluid) and much lower in the small intestine (less than 10,000 bacteria per ml of fluid). Also, the types of bacteria within the small intestine are different to the types of bacteria within the colon. Small intestinal bacterial overgrowth (SIBO) refers to a condition in which abnormally large numbers of bacteria (at least 100,000 bacteria per ml of fluid) are present in the small intestine and the types of bacteria in the small intestine resemble more the bacteria of the colon than the small intestine.

In a study by Qin J et al (*Nature*. 2010 Mar 4;464 (7285):59-65) where the team analysed the top bacteria in order of importance in the microbiome showing

Bacteroides spp. were the most common commensal bacteria, the researchers also showed that patients with IBS have 25 per cent fewer types of bacteria (and therefore genes) present compared to healthy individuals.

The bacteria in the faeces are quite different for ulcerative colitis, IBS, Crohn's disease, and healthy patients. For this reason faecal transplants have been studied as a way of restoring missing genes and the proper balance within the gut.

In a small study at Montefiore Medical Center in New York City, David M. Pinn, M.D. and colleagues took patients where use of dietary modification, probiotics, antibiotics, and/or anti-depressants had failed.

Using Faecal Microbiota Transplants (FMT) they achieved resolved or improved symptoms in 70 percent of the patients with refractory IBS, including abdominal pain (72 percent), bowel habit (69 percent), dyspepsia (67 percent), bloating (50 percent), and flatus (45 percent).

One school of thought suggests that Crohn's and colitis may be treated by attacking the microbes or harmful bacteria that cause the imbalance. Yeasts usually get the blame and anti-yeast diets involving no glucose or cows' dairy, plenty of vegetables and grilled meats and fish, along with anti-yeast treatment (for example, the herb wormwood) and multi-strain probiotics. The late Gerald Green had a lot of success working with patients and several London Medical Schools on this strategy.

According to the American Government website *(http://www.ncbi.nlm.nih.gov/pmc/articles/PMC30025 86/)*, treatment with probiotics does as well as treatment with the steroid mesalamine.

7. Dementia, Alzheimer's

The protein forming plaques in Alzheimer's patients are normally soluble. When the protein folds improperly, it forms amyloid deposits that are associated with brain inflammation. But what causes this inflammation?

UC Davis researchers think they have the answer *(Cell Host & Microbe, July 2012)*. Apparently structures made by some gut bacteria cause a strong immune response. These structures are similar to the myeloid plaques of Alzheimer's. *"Alzheimer's disease may be a case of mistaken identity,"* said Andreas Bäumler, a professor of microbiology and medical immunology.

"Our results suggest that it's the structure of these protein aggregates that matter and that, to the innate immune system, Alzheimer's plaques may look like colonies of bacteria. This would result in the chronic inflammation we see in Alzheimer's disease that damages neurons," Bäumler explained.

Amyloid plaques are the sticky buildup of proteins that accumulate outside nerve cells. They are characteristic of several illnesses, including Alzheimer's disease, Huntington's disease, type 2 diabetes, secondary amyloidosis and prion diseases, like Creutzfeldt-Jakob (the human form of mad cow disease). These diseases all involve marked inflammation at the sites of amyloid deposition, resulting in tissue injury.

The team were not studying Alzheimer's at the time but looking into the causes of inflammation and immune response by gut bacteria.

Importantly, destroying the ability of the gut bacterial proteins to clump together, stopped the formation of Alzheimer's plaques.

The Geriatric Disease Centre at the University of California is looking into bacterial overgrowth in the small intestine and how it is related to memory problems. Normally, the small intestine is free of bacteria but with small intestinal bacterial overgrowth comes the production of large quantities of hydrogen sulphide. In the brain, hydrogen sulphide has been shown to be involved in memory and learning abilities. The team believe that high levels of gut hydrogen sulphide are associated with low levels of brain hydrogen sulphide. And this would impair function.

Research from the University of California, Los Angeles suggests that eating probiotic yogurt can alter your brain function, and with it stress, anxiety, mood and even pain sensitivity. Dr. Kirsten Tillisch of UCLA's School of Medicine found that those who ate probiotic yogurt for a month showed altered brain function, both in resting brain activity and in response to an emotional attention task.

Women were randomly assigned to one of three groups: one that ate a yogurt with live bacterial cultures (containing probiotic strains like *Bifidobacterium animalis*, *Streptococcus thermophiles,* and *Lactobacillus bulgaricus*) twice a day for one month, another that ate a dairy product which contained no living bacteria and another that was given no dairy products.

MRI brain scans and an "emotional faces attention task," were employed. The results showed calmer brains in the probiotic consumers, stronger neural network connections, and clearer decision-making abilities (*Gastroenterology*).

8. Diabetes

"We have demonstrated that people with type-2 diabetes have a high level of pathogens in their intestines," says professor Jun Wang from the University of Copenhagen's Department of Biology and Novo Nordisk Foundation Center for Basic Metabolic Research *(Science Daily, Sept 26th 2012).* In this study, researchers examined the intestinal flora of 345 people from China, of which 171 had type-2 diabetes. Clear biological indicators emerged, and the type-2 subjects had microbiome environments which were more hostile, increasing resistance to drugs. This imbalance in the gut reflected previous findings with Danish subjects showing that people who were 'at risk' of type-2 diabetes had abnormal gut bacterial levels.

That study indicated the typical characteristics of the intestinal flora of type-2 diabetes patients. *"It's a typical flora for someone with a mild form of gastroenteritis"* says Jeroen Raes. *"Now it is also important to include the Western population to see if these markers may be predictors - then the path is open for early diagnostic tests."*

Child research led by Professor Jayne Danska at the *Sick Children's Hospital of the University of Toronto* and Professor Andrew Macpherson in the Clinic for Visceral Surgery and Medicine at the Inselspital and the University of Bern have shown that irregularities in intestinal bacteria may well be causal.

More than 30 years ago Japanese researchers noticed that a strain of NOD laboratory mice tended to get diabetes. Now Danska and Macpherson's teams have shown that the intestinal bacteria, especially in normal male mice, can produce biochemicals and hormones that stop diabetes developing.

In *Nature*, 29 May 2013 *(Gut metagenome in European women with normal, impaired and diabetic glucose control)*, researchers at the Sahlgrenska Academy, University of Gothenburg, Sweden and Chalmers University of Technology, Sweden, have confirmed that women with type-2 diabetes have an altered gut microbiota and lowered levels of bacteria capable of producing sodium butyrate.

On the basis of these findings, the researchers have developed a new predictive model.

And it is possible that **wheat** may have a negatively influencing effect on diabetes too. In November 2013, *(http://www.ncbi.nlm.nih.gov/pmc/articles/PMC38272 56/)*, the following conclusions were made by Mayo Clinic researchers with non-obese diabetic (NOD) mice

1. **GCC-fed (gluten-containing chow fed) NOD mice had the expected high incidence of hyperglycemia (elevated blood sugar) whereas NOD mice fed with a GFC (gluten-free chows) had significantly reduced incidence of hyperglycemia.**

2. **When comparing microbiomes, Bifidobacterium, Tannerella, and Barnesiella species were increased in the intestinal microbiome of GCC mice, where as Akkermansia species was increased in the microbiome of NOD mice fed GFC.**

3. **Both of the gluten-free chows that were evaluated (egg white based, or casein based), significantly reduced the incidence of hyperglycemia.**

It also seems that children who develop type-1 diabetes have different gut flora. *University of Florida* researchers have shown that the variety of bacteria present in a young child's gut is linked to whether it develops type-1 diabetes. Type-1 diabetes has been a medical mystery as there seems little genetic link; less than 15 per cent have another family member with diabetes. Now researchers think the trigger is gut bacteria.

Mark Atkinson, the Professor at the University, looked at Finnish research which first showed a link.

(Finland has a very uniform genetic pool and so is perfect for this sort of research.) *"Diabetes is caused when the body's own immune system destroys insulin-producing cells in the pancreas. It is not clear why."* An unbalanced mix of bacteria in the gut seems to be related in some way. Various theories are suggested – for example, one theory is that the particular mix of bacteria makes the gut wall weak, allowing quite large and complex proteins to cross into the blood stream. The immune system may over-react to them and cause random damage. Another route may be that certain bacteria that are missing would normally suppress inflammation and immune response. University of Florida researchers suggest that this is how poor levels and imbalance of gut bacteria lead to immunological diseases like Crohn's, coeliac disease and even multiple sclerosis. Importantly, in their view, *"the bacterial mix becomes unstable first"*.

9. Heart disease and strokes

April 24, 2013 research *(New England Journal of Medicine)* from Dr. Hazen and his team at the Cleveland Clinic in America shows that phosphatidyl choline, (also called lecithin), a compound in foods like red meat and egg yolks, produces the by-product TMAO when digested. TMAO is known to promote plaque accumulation in the arteries causing heart disease. Explains Dr. Hazen, *"Bacteria that live in our intestines play a role in the digestion of certain types of food to form the compound TMAO, which promotes plaque accumulation in arteries"*. Participants in the study were asked to eat two hard-boiled eggs and take a choline capsule. Results showed that TMAO levels in the blood increased after ingesting the eggs and the capsule. And when participants were given antibiotics to suppress their gut flora, their TMAO levels dropped.

10. Multiple Sclerosis

Researchers at the Max Planck Institute of Neurobiology in Martinsried in Munich, Germany have found evidence that suggests Multiple Sclerosis (MS) is triggered by intestinal flora, bacteria that reside in the gut. Researchers found that gut bacteria seem able to activate T-lymphocytes, then B-lymphocytes in the immune system. These then caused an attack on the myelin sheath in the brain.

Although the research was carried out in mice, researchers feel something similar is likely in humans *(Nature, October 2011)*.

The researchers considered previous research showing active MS lesions have *"inflammatory changes suggestive of a combined attack by autoreactive T- and B-lymphocytes against brain white matter."* While researchers know a lot about the chemical changes that occur in MS, they know little about the causes.

This followed 2010 research from the California Institute of Technology which showed a connection between the microbiome in the gut and the auto-immune disease which attacks both the brain and the spinal column. People sometimes get the disease after bacterial or viral infections, yet the tissues themselves are sterile. This led researchers to look at indirect effects of infections. Mice with no bacteria in their intestines did not get sick. They then introduced a bacterium, Th17; known to cause intestinal inflammation into the mice guts and the mice developed MS symptoms *(July 19-23, Proceedings of the National Academy of Sciences).*

In October 2013, researchers from Weill Cornell Medical College and Rockefeller University discovered the bacterium *Clostridium C. perfringens* type B in a 21-year-old patient suffering from MS and decided to investigate. There are five types of this bacterium. While type-A is normally found in humans, type B and D produce known pathogens and are not.

Both type B and D carry a gene that causes the release of a protoxin pathogen (epsilon), which develops into something much nastier in the intestines of grazing animals. This then moves to the brain, causing damage.

The two types were not thought to occur in humans. Researchers looked for evidence of the toxin in MS patients and found levels of epsilon toxin antibodies ten times higher than those without MS. Stool samples showed that only 23 per cent of MS patients carried the type-A bacterium, compared with 52 per cent of healthy patients.

The significance of this is that type-A seems to compete with the other types. If it is depleted, the others will be dominant *(PLOS ONE, 18 October 2013).*

11. Obesity

Blame it on your bacteria!

A study from the Cedars-Sinai Medical Center in Los Angeles has found that certain types of bacteria in the gut cause it to take more calories from food, therefore leading to weight gain *(Journal of Clinical Endocrinology & Metabolism* 26 March 2013, online issue). The research study used 'breath tests', and a gut bacterium called *Methanobrevibacter smithii* is known to produce most of the methane in the human gut.

Lead researcher Ruchi Mathur says that *"usually bacteria like M. smithii are beneficial because they help extract energy and nutrients from food. But if there is too much M. smithii, it alters the energy balance so as to make the person more likely to put on weight"*

A further study involving animals *(Journal of Proteome Research, Feb 2012)* suggests that bacteria living in the large intestine may play a role in obesity by slowing down the activity of energy-burning brown fat. People have two sorts of fat, brown and white. White is typically a store, and lies around the waist. Brown fat however burns calories when stimulated and young and thin people have more brown than white fat. Researchers, from Imperial College, London, UK, and the Nestlé Research Centre in Lausanne, Switzerland found that regular mice with normal gut microbiomes burned brown fat slower than the mice that had no bacteria in their intestines. Males burned fat more slowly than females.

Research from a group jointly led by Oluf Pederson of the University of Copenhagen *(Nature online: 10.1038/Nature12506, Le Chatelier, Aug 23, 2013)* has suggested that there are links between the bacteria in the gut and medical complications related to obesity. The controlling factor seems to be diversity. Healthy flora contain a diversity of bacteria not found in people with medical conditions.

Pederson is part of the international consortium *MetaHIT*, which includes the research group of Jeroen Raes (VIB/Vrije Universiteit Brussel). They compared the flora of 169 obese Danes with 123 non-obese Danes. The researchers observed that the group with less diverse flora in their gut were more prone to obesity and inflammation. However, there were some obese people with a rich diversity of flora. Nevertheless, the poorer flora were more prevalent in the obese group and were linked with adiposity, insulin resistance, chronic inflammation and more cardiovascular complications. Jeroen Raes said, *"This is an amazing result with possibly enormous implications for the treatment and even prevention of the greatest public health issue of our time. But we are not there yet, now we need studies in which we can monitor people for a longer period. We want to perform these types of long-term studies together with the 'Vlaams Darmflora Project' (Flemish Gut Flora Project), which is only possible thanks to the selfless efforts of thousands of Flemish residents."*

Researchers believe 23 per cent of the population has

a poor diversity of bacteria in their microbiome. And, it seems, leaner people have a more diverse microbiome.

Perhaps the most bizarre research study in this book comes from Washington University in St Louis where Dr. Jeffrey I Gordon and his team took human twins, where one was fat and the other thin. Having extracted the microbiome, they then gave the bacteria to identical mice. And guess what happened? Yup. The mice getting the fat guy's bacteria got fat, and the mice with the thin guy's bacteria got thin.

Now before all you chubbies reading this breathe a self-centred sigh of relief, you need to know about the rest of the study. Here the fat and thin mice were put in the same cage, and all fed a low-fat diet. Mice also eat one another's droppings. So in the end they all had the same gut bacteria, and with their low-fat diet, they all became thin. Thin bacteria dominate fat ones. So you've all got a chance.

For the final part of the study, the group put the fat mice together with the thin ones but this time offered two types of food, equivalent to the good or bad diets prevalent in the West. The fat mice that ate food high in fat and low in fruits and vegetables kept the gut bacteria from the fat twin, remaining fat. The thin twins' gut bacteria took over only when the mice ate pellets that were rich in fruits and vegetables and low in fat.

So, ultimately, you are what you feed your bacteria.

In quite a few years' time, they may have isolated thin people's bacteria (tpb) and fat people may be given probiotic tbp pills. But you will of course have to eat lots of fruit and vegetables and quit the bad foods.

I did not write this on April 1st.

12. Parkinson's

A common bacterial infection may contribute to Parkinson's disease (PD) risk, according to research published in the *European Journal of Neurology,* April 2012. The bacterium, *Helicobacter pylori*, is ever present in our bodies but, when in excess, it is more commonly associated with stomach problems, including ulcers and occasionally stomach cancer. (Note stomach, not large intestine). The large population study showed that, out of 3,489 people who eventually developed Parkinson's, 138 of them, or 3.9 percent, had been treated for *H. pylori*. In the control group, 2.9 percent had been treated for *H. pylori*.

Researchers have long been puzzled as to why many people with Parkinson's have a history of stomach problems, such as ulcers, prior to developing Parkinson's. The study revealed a 46 percent increase in the likelihood of developing Parkinson's if the person had been treated for *H. pylori* at least five years prior.

The study used two large Danish databases, one full of information regarding drug prescriptions and one of medical records. For every person with Parkinson's identified, Dr. Ritz and colleagues randomly selected five controls without Parkinson's, of the same sex and age. They then looked for a connection between the prescription of drugs that treat *H. pylori* and the eventual clinical diagnosis of Parkinson's five years later.

So, did *Helicobacter pylori* cause the Parkinson's or was it the drugs affecting the microbiome?

There's no answer to this question, but a leaky gut may also be causal.

Dr. Ali Keshavarzian, a Gastroenterologist at Rush Medical Center, Chicago, became involved in Parkinson's when his sister developed the disease. At a seminar he learned how laboratory research showed that alcohol, which can cause gastrointestinal permeability (or gut leakiness), can also cause brain damage similar to Parkinson's disease. If lipopolysaccharide (LPS), a toxin produced by certain intestinal bacteria, also escaped, the damage to the brain lasted longer.

"We know that stress, like alcohol, can cause the gut to leak. What if stress causes leaks that let LPS into the body? A person would have to have a genetic susceptibility for the disease, but the LPS leakage might be the trigger for Parkinson's."

Six years after the hypothesis, clinical trial results (May 2012) linked LPS leaking out of the intestine with a chain of nerve-cell changes that move to the brain and become Parkinson's disease.

* *

Further References

1. Bu LN, Chang MH, Ni YH, Chen HL, Cheng CC: Lactobacillus casei rhamnosus Lcr35 in children with chronic constipation. *Pediatr Int* 2007, 49:485-490.

2. Picard C, Fioramonti J, Francois A, Robinson T, Neant F, Matuchansky C: Review article: bifidobacteria as probiotic agents – physiological effects and clinical benefits. *Aliment Pharmacol Ther* 2005, 22:495-512.

3. Bouvier M, *et al.*: Effects of consumption of a milk fermented by the probiotic B. animalis DN-173 010 on colonic transit time in healthy humans. *Bioscience and microflora* 2001, 20:43-48.

4. Marteau P, Cuillerier E, Meance S, Gerhardt MF, Myara A, Bouvier M, Bouley C, Tondu F, Bommelaer G, Grimaud JC: Bifidobacterium animalis strain DN-173 010 shortens the colonic transit time in healthy women: a double-blind, randomized, controlled study. *Aliment Pharmacol Ther* 2002, 16:587-593.

5. Koebnick C, Wagner I, Leitzmann P, Stern U, Zunft HJ: Probiotic beverage containing Lactobacillus casei Shirota improves gastrointestinal symptoms in patients with chronic constipation. *Can J Gastroenterol* 2003, 17:655-659.

6. Banaszkiewicz A, Szajewska H: Ineffectiveness of Lactobacillus GG as an adjunct to lactulose for the treatment of constipation in children: a double-blind, placebo-controlled randomized trial. *J Pediatr* 2005, 146:364-369.

7. Meance S, Turchet P: A fermented milk with a Bifidobacterium probiotic Strain DN-173 010 shortened oro-fecal gut transit time in elderly. Microb Ecol Health Dis 2001, 13:217-222.

CHAPTER 15
THE BOTTOM LINE

We each represent a triumph of evolution – a sophisticated ecosystem of 100 trillion cells and 100,000 genes controlling our mental and physical abilities. The direction of this ecosystem lies with the genes at its heart, three-quarters of which are not ours but those of our symbiotic bacteria.

Can anybody now doubt that the loss of 'good bacteria', the loss of diversity, the over-expression of harmful bacteria, microbes and parsites, results in an imbalanced microbiome and puts our health – both physical and mental - at risk?

The aim of this short book was simply to bring this 'secret' to the masses. As I said at the outset, it's a secret that I knew in 2004, but seems, even today, to elude many in the medical profession.

I talked of the 'inconvenient truth'. That a microbiome that becomes sick leads to a host that becomes sick. And a host cannot become well again until their microbiome is returned to health? The 'inconvenient truth' is that the very people given the job of protecting our health, have been making matters worse. They have encouraged:

- A preoccupation with eradicating 'germs',

pasteurisation, irradiation, even the outright banning of some 'bacteria-containing' foods we have always thrived on. This is clearly misguided.

- A lax policy on pesticides and herbicides, and a lack of independent regulation on GMO foods both directly and indirectly. This threatens our friendly bacteria, and the messages, proteins, enzymes and helpful compounds they provide us with.

- The widespread use of cocktails of prescription drugs and antibiotics (Biota = life, so antibiotics = anti-life). These provoke a direct attack on the existence of our essential bacteria.

- Treating gut problems with drugs, which clearly make matters worse. (When there are natural remedies that are both effective and restore balance to the ecosystem.)

- A movement to refined food, fast food, high sugar drinks, and this has come at a clear cost to our health. The benefits of vegetables, fruits and a high fibre diet to grow a strong microbiome have never been explained to people.

The coming paradigm shift in health treatment

There are some interesting issues worthy of further debate. For example, perhaps the medical profession has been treating the wrong body? Maybe they would get better results if they treated the one with 93 trillion cells not the one with 7 trillion?

There is no doubt that research is going to gather pace. The growth of our knowledge about our personal ecosystems is going to be huge. This is unstoppable.

But. Are we going to witness the usual medical extremes? Ignore or embrace?

Perhaps we will just see the core of Western medical dogma continuing with their drugs as if nothing was happening.

Or will we see a genuine paradigm shift in health treatment that, in truth, this new knowledge should bring?

And then, will we witness a rush to embrace faecal transplants? If so, will the 'embrace' doctors want to sort out the health of the microbiome first; or will the 'ignore' doctors continue to use their traditional methods then correct the gut microbiome afterwards?

Will faecal transplants be regulated as treatments? Or can anyone offer them? Will we see a rush to open private clinics – the new 'alternative treatment' for all ills? Will there be 'best practice'?

Playing with genetics

Technically, the truth is that we are in danger of playing with the genome by introducing DNA into the body; and research already shows that this DNA can be taken up by the host.

If the 'super probiotic' is launched, will just any company be to allowed do this? After all, the super probiotic contains genetic material that can control not just your health, but your mental attitude. The gut microbiome project people are collecting samples from thousands of people, right now. What might they or others do with this genetic material?

At the moment, the whole area of probiotics is almost unregulated – anybody can seemingly just launch one. Some have 3 billion a pill; others shout that they have 60 billion. But when people understand that it is diversity not volume that matters, will we be seeing probiotics with 200 or 300 strains? Think of all that genetic material being introduced into your ecosystem. Surely, not just any old vitamin company is going to be allowed to sell this? But who will regulate it? Health Authorities? With their past close involvement with Big Pharma and bias, how could we be sure that we really did receive all the bacteria we needed?

Already psychiatrists are talking about using faecal transplants on the mentally ill. Will any line be drawn over who is or is not 'treated'? As our knowledge about specific bacteria and their effects increases, will there be moves to treat not just depression and Parkinson's but perhaps the mentally unstable, even criminals?

Will there be attempts to provide babies with super probiotics soon after birth to kick-start their immune system if they are born by Caesarian?

Where will this lead? To different super probiotics for children that can lead to calmer adults? Will certain bacteria be on a restricted list? "This bacterium will make you aggressive" - Great if you are in the army, banned if you are an Olympic boxer.

While this whole area is full of potential, some of the issues are almost Orwellian.

Microbiologists can now predict with 90 per cent accuracy, just from your faeces, whether you are lean or fat, whether you have diabetes, or MS. And what illness you are at risk of developing. This brings a whole new focus to the concept of prevention. Catch the problem early and change your microbiome balance. Who needs drugs?

If you become ill, bring on the faecal transplant or super probiotic. Who needs surgery?

The human personal ecosystem

Humans have been colonised by bacteria for a very, very long time. And the principle of the 'survival of the fittest' dictates that these bacteria in humans today are the best at what they do; they are still with us because they are extraordinarily helpful to us. They participate in our biochemistry, our physiology and our psychology. They provide an overwhelming array of cells and genes, proteins and bioactive compounds, messages and commands.

Do we control their lives? Or do they control ours?

Clearly, we don't treat them right; we threaten their very existence – and, thus, ours too.

This is a complex but vitally important, personal ecosystem.

You cannot survive without its essential functions. Disturb the natural balance at your peril. Protect yourself by protecting it with the foods you eat and your lifestyle. Treat them well; provide the things they like; avoid the poisons (for that's what they are).

And top up your microbiome whenever you think it may have been compromised.

Above all, remember it is there with you all the time, relying on you to look after it. It's the secret source of your good health.

CANCERactive

CANCERactive is a UK Registered Charity (No. 1102413). Its aims, as agreed with the Charities Commission, are 'to inform and support' cancer patients and to provide 'research' into treatments.

CANCERactive Mission

The aim of the charity is to provide information, not just on orthodox cancer treatments but on complementary and new, alternative therapies allowing people to make more informed personal choices and so increase their personal odds of survival.

The Trustees of the charity have found that the aim of conducting original research requires funding out of keeping with the funds raised. However, much quality research is available around the world and is not fully communicated to cancer patients. We will fulfill our mission in the 'research' area by making sure people can easily access scientific research that is particularly relevant to personal health.

CANCERactive provides the information in a number of ways:

1. A 3600 page website (www.canceractive.com)

2. A unique, free magazine called Integrated Cancer and Oncology News (**icon**) available in 640 hospitals, cancer clinics, health centres and libraries in the UK.

3. Downloadable prevention leaflets

4. Catherine Corners in Chichester, the Wirral, Hull and Kenilworth.

5. A series of books compiled by Chris Woollams

6. A second patient support website (www.canceractivepatientgroup.com)

Readers should note that:

1. All books are compiled and written for CANCERactive by Chris Woollams from information on the website and contained in the research centre Cancer Watch.

2. Books include:

The Tree of Life (now The Rainbow Diet and how it can help you beat cancer)

Everything you need to know to help you beat cancer

Cancer - your first 15 steps

Oestrogen - the killer in our midst

Conventional Cancer Cures - what's the alternative ?

The Secret Source of Your Good Health (Published by Health Issues)

Helpful websites

CANCERactive: www.canceractive.com
Patient group: www.canceractivepatientgroup.com
Health Issues: www.ournaturalselection.com
All illnesses: www.chriswoollamshealthline.com
www.chriswoollamshealthwatch.com

CANCERactive has neither distribution facilities, nor a sales operation. The Trustees of CANCERactive have appointed Health Issues Ltd as the sole distributor for all CANCERactive published books and **i c o n** magazine in the UK, USA and Europe.